"Proof that I do *not* need another vet getting in my way," she said aloud, the defiant declaration sailing from her lips only moments before her foot slipped out from under her.

Flying backward, she squeezed her eyes shut and braced for impact. Except...instead of slamming onto the ground, she was pulled out of thin air by... *something*.

A guardian angel? She had read about such unseen interventions in moments of peril. But as she opened her eyes and peered downward, the lightly tanned, muscular arms wrapped around her waist looked anything but ghostlike. The arms remained in place for several moments—long enough for her to become fully aware of the body they were attached to. She couldn't see it yet, but she could feel its warmth and strength bolstering her up from behind.

"You good?" a male voice asked with an Australian accent so deep and sexy that it made her male Vermont counterparts sound like Pee Wee Herman.

Dear Reader,

This book will always have a special place in my heart. Not only because of my profound love for horses, but because I've witnessed firsthand the incredible dedication of the veterinarians—both men and women—who care for these magnificent animals. It's not an easy job (picture emergency calls in the middle of the night and in the dead of winter...), but when it comes to the health and welfare of horses, "can't do" is not a phrase in their vocabulary.

In *A Date with Her Rival*, things get off to a bumpy start when equine veterinarian Maya finds a handsome new colleague, Cal, suddenly in her midst. She has her reasons for preferring to go it alone, both personally and professionally, just as he has his reasons for never staying in one place for too long.

But the deep compassion that they share for horses brings them closer and makes them realize they might just want the same things in life...including a future together.

I truly enjoyed writing this book and helping Maya and Cal find the happily-ever-after they both deserve. I hope you enjoy their story as well!

Tessa

A DATE WITH HER RIVAL

TESSA SCOTT

MEDICAL ROMANCE

If you purchased this book without a cover you should be aware that this book is stolen property. It was reported as "unsold and destroyed" to the publisher, and neither the author nor the publisher has received any payment for this "stripped book."

Recycling programs for this product may not exist in your area.

ISBN-13: 978-1-335-99325-0

A Date with Her Rival

Copyright © 2025 by Tessa Scott

All rights reserved. No part of this book may be used or reproduced in any manner whatsoever without written permission.

Without limiting the author's and publisher's exclusive rights, any unauthorized use of this publication to train generative artificial intelligence (AI) technologies is expressly prohibited.

This is a work of fiction. Names, characters, places and incidents are either the product of the author's imagination or are used fictitiously. Any resemblance to actual persons, living or dead, businesses, companies, events or locales is entirely coincidental.

For questions and comments about the quality of this book, please contact us at CustomerService@Harlequin.com.

TM and ® are trademarks of Harlequin Enterprises ULC.

Harlequin Enterprises ULC
22 Adelaide St. West, 41st Floor
Toronto, Ontario M5H 4E3, Canada
www.Harlequin.com

HarperCollins Publishers
Macken House, 39/40 Mayor Street Upper,
Dublin 1, D01 C9W8, Ireland
www.HarperCollins.com

Printed in U.S.A.

Tessa Scott is a lover of animals, nature and happily-ever-afters. She lives in Northeast Connecticut surrounded by lots of trees, wildlife and a menagerie of pets. A copywriter by day, she enjoys that magical moment when the characters she creates come to life and help take the story in new and exciting directions.

Books by Tessa Scott

Healing the Baby Surgeon's Heart

Visit the Author Profile page at Harlequin.com.

In memory of Piper, my sweet, beautiful boy who was with me for twenty-eight years and is now galloping through meadows beyond the Rainbow Bridge.
Until we meet again.

CHAPTER ONE

MAYA EVANS STARED wide-eyed at her dad, hoping that she had misheard him. "You didn't just say you hired another vet."

He gingerly raised his thick, gray eyebrows, as though bracing for further objections. *"Temporarily,"* he emphasized. "Just long enough for you to get fully back on your feet."

Maya looked down at her sturdy work boots, which were planted firmly on the dirt-trodden ground. She looked back up at her father as if to say, *I'm good, but thanks for checking!*

He let out a long sigh, followed by a begrudging smile. "You're more stubborn than a mule. Even Betty looks like a cream puff next to you," he said, referring to a recent patient who was, in fact, a mule. The comparison slightly amused Maya, and she felt the corners of her lips curve upward. But then, reality set in and the smile melted away.

The last time her dad had brought another vet on board their practice, it had ended in heartbreak. Not only for herself, but also for her eight-year-old son, Jeremy. What had started as a professional relationship with Dr. Max Shepard had turned into a romantic one, and when Max decided to relocate to

Texas for a prestigious veterinary college teaching position, both she and Jeremy, who had come to see him as a surrogate father, were devastated.

Of course, her father was hiring a temporary vet, not a potential romantic interest for her. For all she knew, the doctor was female. *But that's not the point.* He should have consulted her first. Yes, he had started Northern Vermont Equine Associates back when she was still in diapers and had built it from the ground up, but now he was semiretired, with full retirement expected in the very near future. Which meant the brunt of the burgeoning practice fell on her increasingly weary shoulders. So shouldn't she have an active say in any hiring decisions, temporary or otherwise?

"I like to work alone, Dad," she said quietly.

"I know you do, Maya," he said with empathy in his eyes that indicated he knew this wasn't just about her streak of independence. "But your arm is still in a cast, and given that you wince every time you turn, I'm going to assume those cracked ribs still have some healing left as well." He paused. "Am I right?"

As if on cue, her left side pinched as she drew in a deep breath. "I can still do my job."

"It's your job that got you injured in the first place—remember?"

Maya pursed her lips in silent acknowledgement. It was her fault, and hers alone, that Roofus the giant Clydesdale had kicked her like an errant tumbleweed when she'd been treating his hoof abscess several weeks ago. He had *seemed* to be fully under the effects of a mild sedation, still standing as needed for the procedure, his lower lip drooping and eyelids half closed.

But one clamp of the hoof pincers to find the sensitive area hiding the abscess, and Roofus had rustled up enough lingering adrenaline to promptly send Maya flying across the matted floor of the clinic. She shuddered at the recollection of ending up in a heap several feet away, struggling to breathe as immense pain had gripped her side and shot through her left forearm.

Shake it off. A few deep breaths, and Maya was back in the present, searing pain replaced with residual discomfort at the still-sensitive sites of her injuries.

"Dad, you know this is just part of being an equine vet. How many times over the years did you end up bruised and battered from a particularly difficult client?"

"Are you talking the horses, or their pain-in-the-butt owners?" he asked with a grin.

Maya shook her head and reluctantly chuckled. If anyone knew the highs and lows of life as a horse veterinarian, it was her dad. She couldn't remember a time when he hadn't been tending to whinnying, four-legged patients for a living, but arthritis in both of his hands had made it increasingly difficult to perform even the most basic of equine care.

"Look, Maya. At some point, we're going to need to bring another vet on board. We're at capacity right now with our current clients, and it seems like every week we're getting calls for potential new ones. I've had to ask Maria to put them on a waiting list," he said, referring to their part-time business manager.

Maya's eyes flashed with surprise and concern. "Seriously?"

"Yes. I haven't said anything to you, because I know you don't like to turn down anyone needing help for their horse. And I did instruct Maria to give them the names of other vets in the area. But we're no longer a two-person team. More like one and one-eighth person team, given the limited hours I can put in. And by the end of the year, I plan to be fully retired." He pushed out a smile. "Not that I don't love Vermont winters, but I don't think my creaky, old hips can take another season of wading through two feet of snow to get to a patient out in the field."

Maya's face softened with understanding. "I know. And believe me, I don't want you to have to deal with another tough winter. You should instead be on the beach someplace warm, sipping on margaritas and working on a tan."

Her father grinned. "Actually, I plan to be in my mountain chalet right here in Maplewood, sipping on hot cocoa in front of a roaring fire. The only difference is I won't be heading out at midnight in a snowstorm to help deliver a foal."

Maya smiled, even though the mere thought of

frigid January temperatures triggered a brief shiver under her lightweight fall jacket. "That's where I come in."

His face relaxed, as though relieved to see that Maya was slowly coming around to the idea of temporary help. "I realize it will take some time to find a vet that you're comfortable with bringing on board permanently, but in the meantime, we have someone to help pick up the slack for two months. That's all this is. Think of it as buying some time while you start searching for someone who *you* want to bring on board full-time. After all, the practice will be fully yours soon enough."

Maya's eyes scanned the panoramic scenery as she and her dad stood outside the main barn. Mid-September in Vermont was a feast for the eyes, with the rolling mountains in the background awash with the brilliant red, orange and golden swatches of autumn. But in only a few months, the colorful leaves would be dropping from the trees, signaling the arrival of winter—and the official passing of the torch with her dad's inevitable retirement.

It wasn't that she didn't realize the practice was too busy to handle all on her own. That was a no-brainer. But working in tandem with another vet meant gelling with them on multiple levels. It wasn't enough that they came fully equipped with an expert veterinary skill set. Did they also share her compassion and love for horses? Which would seem like a given but—in the same vein as medical doctors devoid of a bedside manner—wasn't always the case. Would they respect that she had two main priorities at this point in her life—her young son and the horses in her care—and everything else came third?

She could go on and on in her thoughts...but the bottom line was she *did* need an extra set of hands. Which meant she had to accept the current game plan, like it or not.

Maya turned to her father. "So, what can you tell me about this temporary hire?" Just saying the word *temporary* made her feel at least a *little* better, given that it implied she had some control over future events.

"Well, I fully vetted him." He paused for effect. "No pun intended. I think you'll like him."

Him. So it was a male vet, not too surprising given there was a fifty-fifty chance of that being the case.

"And he's Australian."

Maya did a double take. "Australian? And he's here in Vermont?" Though she couldn't picture a more perfect place to live than in the quintessential New England town of Maplewood, with its vibrant four seasons and yesteryear charm...she also couldn't imagine it registered on any map found in the pocket of a global traveler.

"He said he prefers to not stay in any one place too long, so he picks up veterinary gigs wherever the wind takes him."

Maya had to force her gaping mouth to close.

Only then could she reply, her voice rising with each word. "Wherever the wind takes him?"

"I think that's how he described it." Her father shifted his weight from one leg to the other, as though realizing he was quickly losing ground with his dubious daughter. "Think of it as... I don't know...like a traveling nurse. Only in this case, he's a traveling horse vet."

Maya narrowed her eyes. "That sounds *very* fishy to me. You sure he's not a fugitive pretending to be a vet?"

Her father chuckled. "I'm sure. His credentials all checked out, and I even had him weigh in on a few cases while he was here. I have to say, I was quite impressed."

Maya's disbelief was snowballing. "When did all of this happen?"

"This morning. I thought you'd be here, but you had that emergency colic case in Cantonville. He recently finished a gig in California, and was looking for something on the East Coast. We had a phone interview a few days ago that went really well, so he flew in for an in-person interview. I had planned to loop you in sooner, but I know how busy you've been and everything happened so fast." He paused, eyes probing hers as though trying to land on what to say next. "He, uh, reminded me a bit of Crocodile Dundee."

Maya scrunched her lips together. If her dad thought he was sweetening the pot with this comparison, he was way off the mark. "There were no Australian vets applying for the job who could double for Chris Hemsworth?"

Her father looked perplexed. "Who?"

She smiled and shook her head. "Never mind." There were already so many red flags popping up at every turn that all she could do was accept the situation and take solace in the fact that it was a short-term solution. "When does he start?"

"Should be any day. He's looking for a place to rent while he's here, and once that's taken care of, he'll be reporting for duty."

"Can't wait," Maya deadpanned.

Her dad smiled warily. "Try not to bite off his head."

Maya pointed to herself with mock indignation. "Me?"

It was early dusk when Maya returned to the main barn. She pulled her phone out of her back jeans pocket and called Clara, the trusty caregiver who looked after Jeremy while she was at work. "I'll be home in about twenty minutes," she said, smiling as she received a comforting update about her son. He was playing with their dog, Rusty, after finishing his school homework.

She was about to ask Clara to pass the phone to Jeremy, then thought better of it. He was having fun with Rusty, just as a young boy should. There was no need to pull him away from that.

Maya's smile wavered as she thought about how

much he'd already been through in his short lifetime. At the tender age of three, he had lost his father, George. Even now, the thought of her late husband pried open the floodgate to bittersweet memories. A fellow horse vet in the family practice, George had died tragically in a car accident on the way to an emergency call.

It hadn't been easy picking up the pieces after his death, but Maya had been determined to stay strong for both of them. And then, just over two years ago, Max came onto the scene...slowly working his way into both her heart and Jeremy's.

Maya winced. She knew how that story ended, too, and wasn't about to go there again in her thoughts.

"Maya?"

Carla's voice brought her back to the present.

"I'm sorry," Maya said into the phone. "Did you say something?"

"I just wasn't sure if there was something else you needed to tell me."

"Oh—no, I don't think so." Her smile slowly returned. "I'll see you guys in a little bit."

Maya ended the call, acknowledging to herself once again how lucky she was to have found Carla. In her mid-fifties and exuding natural warmth and nurturing, Carla lived in a cozy apartment above the garage on Maya's ten-acre property. It was a mutually beneficial arrangement, with Carla enjoying rent-free housing in exchange for keeping a watchful eye on Jeremy while Maya was at work.

And that could pretty much be any time, and often with little notice. The life of a horse vet promised many things, but working a nine-to-five job was not one of them. At least not with a smaller practice that provided twenty-four seven emergency service for its clients spread out over a fifty-mile radius.

After doling out grain and filling water buckets for the five horses currently receiving on-site care, Maya sighed wearily at the realization that there were no hay bales available in the barn aisle. Jenna, the local horse-loving teen who worked part-time after school at the clinic, normally pulled a few bales down from the loft before heading out for the night. Maya nodded to herself and murmured, "Oh, that's right," as she vaguely recalled Maria mentioning that Jenna had called in sick.

Placing the hand of her cast-free arm on the ladder, she looked up at the twelve wooden rungs that ascended vertically into the dark loft opening. It was a simple enough task to make the climb and throw down a couple of bales—at least it was with two good arms and pain-free ribs. Still, she could do this. She *had* to do this.

Here goes nothing. She drew in a deep breath for good measure. Grabbing onto the closest ladder rung with her right hand, she began the climb, carefully balancing with her left hand as well. There was a strange pulling sensation in her left forearm as she closed her hand around the ladder rungs, but that was to be expected. Though her radius was close to fully healed, the muscles surrounding it were atrophied from limited use.

A few more steps up the ladder and she was in the loft area, surrounded by rows of hay bales stacked six deep. She removed the metal hay pull that hung on the wall, yanked down three bales with her good arm, then dragged them to the loft opening and pushed them through.

Each landed with a muffled thud, followed by anxious whinnying that rumbled through the barn.

"Hang on, guys," she called out as she started her descent down the ladder. "Dinner's coming!"

This is easier than I expected, she thought as she lowered herself from one rung to the next, her right hand singularly grasping the side rail to steady herself. "Proof that I do *not* need another vet getting in my way," she said aloud, the defiant declaration sailing from her lips only moments before her foot slipped out from under her.

Grabbing the nearest rung with both hands, she yelped as pain shot through her left arm. Logic told her to hang on anyway, but in the split second that she had to commit to a course of action, logic was replaced with panic.

Flying backward, she squeezed her eyes shut and braced for impact. Except…instead of slamming onto the ground, she was pulled out of thin air by… *something*.

A guardian angel? She had read about such unseen interventions in moments of peril. But as she opened her eyes and peered downward, the lightly tanned, muscular arms wrapped around her waist looked anything but ghostlike. The arms remained in place for several moments—long enough for her to become fully aware of the body they were attached to. She couldn't *see* the body yet, but she could feel its warmth and strength bolstering her up from behind.

"You good?" a male voice asked with an Australian accent so deep and sexy that it made her male Vermont counterparts sound like Pee-wee Herman.

Maya swallowed hard and winced, then slowly turned around, nearly shuddering as her eyes fell upon the man who had just spared her from more broken bones. With greenish-blue eyes, a chiseled jawline and dark blond hair that skimmed his shoulders, his vibe was definitely more Chris Hemsworth than Crocodile Dundee—and with smoldering good looks that were uniquely his own.

"Sorry," he said as he let go of her waist, a subtly mischievous grin on his face. "I didn't mean to get in your way."

Maya grimaced sheepishly. "Oh…you heard that…"

His grin widened. "No worries. It's the kind of thing I would've said myself, to be honest." He held out his hand. "Cal Parker."

"Maya Evans," she replied, shaking his hand

while simultaneously trying to steady herself. Whether from the adrenaline rush that accompanied her fall, or the shock of landing in the arms of a handsome stranger, she was feeling more than a little disoriented. "You must be the vet that my dad hired this morning."

He nodded. "That would be me."

"I wasn't expecting you for a few more days, but glad you showed up early." Maya cocked her head in the direction of her cast-covered arm. "Another broken bone, and I'd be out of the game for good."

"Glad I remembered how to catch," Cal said, seeming to stop just short of a wink. "It can be hard enough doing this job with full mobility. I can only imagine what it's like with an arm that's out of commission."

"Well, hopefully not for much longer. My cast comes off in a few weeks."

"I like the color," Cal said as he glanced at the turquoise moldable wrap covering the hard cast.

Thanks, it matches your eyes.

Luckily, Maya only *thought* this reply—but even that was disturbing to her.

Cal nodded to her midsection. "And the ribs?"

"Guess my father really filled you in," Maya said, nearly squirming inside as his intense gaze worked its way back up from her waist. *Gulp.*

"He just told me about the accident you had, that's all. But sounds like you're healing up nicely."

Maya was tempted to say more, if for no other reason than to hear Cal reply in his sexy accent. Heck, he could recite the alphabet right now, and she'd be hanging on every letter.

Get a grip on yourself, girl!

Maya's shoulders twinged slightly, jolted by her inner admonishment. But it was the wake-up call that she needed.

"Are you still looking for a place to stay?" she asked, doing her best to get back to all business.

"I already found one this afternoon—a cabin at the base of Hickory Mountain. The owner lives in New York and uses it during ski season, but he's traveling overseas until late January." He paused to smile, revealing a slight dimple in his left cheek. "So I guess it's home for me for the next couple of months."

Maya forced a smile of her own, in part to keep her mouth from blurting out a less-than-friendly question. After all, asking Cal whether he couldn't commit to a permanent job because he was on the lam from the law *probably* wasn't the best way to get their working relationship off the ground.

"That's a beautiful area," she finally said. "And the skiing come winter is great. Do you ski?"

"On water," Cal said with a slight grin. "Although I'm always up for a new challenge."

"Hmm. I'm sure you are."

Cal's eyes widened at her pointed barb, but it had slipped out of her mouth before she had a chance to clamp down on her cynical thoughts. But could he blame her? After all, it was hard—make that *impossible*—not to picture him eagerly chasing down a new two-legged filly each time he breezed into a new gig. Although, with his rugged good looks and oh-so-smooth bonhomie, most of the fillies no doubt willingly galloped his way, no chase needed. But there was always an exception to the rule, and Maya was determined to be the one woman who would *not* succumb to his charms. *Nope. Not me.*

"Did you come by to tell my dad that you found a place? He's only here until noon most days, so he's back home for the night."

"I came to check on Baxter, actually."

Maya raised an eyebrow. "Oh...?"

"Not sure if your dad mentioned this to you, but when I came by for the interview this morning, he asked me to weigh in on some of the tough cases you're working on."

Maya bristled. It already felt like Cal was encroaching on her territory, especially after she was so used to working alone. Yes, she needed help... but did it have to be this sudden? Realizing she was possibly being...*oh, just a tad bit*...unreasonable, Maya did her best to drop down her guard a notch.

Cal intensified his gaze on her and squinted, as though sizing up her apprehension. It was a by-product of working around horses, Maya thought to herself. One couldn't help but learn to read the slightest shifts in body language, just like equines did. And Cal was reading her now.

"I probably should have given you a heads-up that I was coming by," he said.

Maya quietly caught her breath. "That's okay." She held up her left arm. "It's good that you did—remember?"

There was an earnestness in Cal's eyes that made her dial down her distrust of the situation. *Give him a chance*, she inwardly insisted, before nodding toward a stall at the front of the barn. "Let's go see Baxter."

For someone used to casually rolling into new situations without so much as the blink of an eye...*both* of Cal's eyes were now uncharacteristically working overtime. How could they not, when the most beautiful woman he'd ever seen was smack-dab in front of him?

As he followed her to the stall, Maya briefly looked back and narrowed her eyes at him as if to say *Are you looking at my butt?*

Heck, yeah, he silently acknowledged. But the gentleman in him was not about to give away as much. Instead, he did his best I'm just moseying on along impression, looking to the left and then the right, and stopping himself just short of breaking out into nonchalant whistling. No need to be *too* obvious in covering his tracks.

Maya turned to face forward again, but not before Cal caught a glimpse of a slight smile on her beguiling face. Or maybe it was a grimace, and he only imagined that the curve of her lips faced upward instead of down.

Either way, once he was out of her eyesight, *his* eyes wasted no time picking up where they had left off. Maya was petite, about five foot two, he reckoned, but she had enough lean curves to fill out her tight jeans in all the right places. Her dark ash-brown hair tumbled down her back, bouncing with every determined step.

In fact, he couldn't recall ever seeing someone of her diminutive size covering ground at such a rapid pace. He quickened his own step to keep up, prompting several horses to stick their heads out over the stall gates as he whizzed by, side-eying him as if to say, *No trotting in the barn.*

Maya entered Baxter's stall and held the gate open for Cal.

"Hi, sweetie," she said to Baxter, a compact, dark bay Morgan, as she scratched him under the chin and nuzzled him affectionately. Cal watched, mesmerized, wishing he could instantly grow a tail and pointed ears so he could receive some of Maya's nuzzles as well.

When she turned to him, her light gray eyes latching onto his, he patted Baxter on the withers. Anything to avoid looking like a fool with a too-obvious stare back.

"So, as I imagine my dad must have told you, Baxter's been here for just over a week with pastern dermatitis that refuses to heal."

Given that Maya seemed more than a little leery of his presence, Cal knew he had to find a way to pass muster with her. Forget about a flirty smile, which he could tell would be about as warmly received on her end as a *Titanic*-sized iceberg. Rather, he needed to prove his equine veterinary chops—and fast.

Right...pastern dermatitis, he repeated inwardly as a quick refresher.

He knew that the oozing, crusty skin condition, also known by no fewer than a half dozen other names, such as mud fever and dew poisoning, had a variety of causes, including bacteria, fungus or excessive moisture in the back pastern area just above the hoof. It typically cleared up quickly with topical treatment, but every once in a while, there was a stubborn case that defied the norm.

"We've tried everything," Maya said. "Antibiotic and steroid creams, zinc oxide cream, a silver antibacterial sock..."

Cal pulled a small jar out of his jacket pocket—the reason for his unannounced visit in the first place. "Triple Strength Healing Clay, found in every horse barn and veterinary clinic in Australia. Works wonders for pastern dermatitis. I can't tell you *why* it does when all these expensive pharmaceutical solutions fail...but sometimes it's the old farmers' remedies that work best."

Maya glanced at the jar, looking less than sold on its merits. "We've already tried a clay drying paste that helped for a couple of days, before the area started oozing again."

Cal flashed a half-smile. "Ahh...but was it clay from Lake Mungo in New South Wales?"

She stared at him unblinkingly. "No."

Well, she didn't inherit her dad's warmth, that's for sure, Cal thought ruefully as he handed her the jar. "Give this a try." He waited for her to reply, then decided to take matters into his own hands. Removing disposable gloves from his jacket pocket, he snapped them on and bent down, lifting Baxter's infected leg. "I'll put some on him now."

Maya opened the jar and bent down so that it was within Cal's reach. As her lightly perfumed hair swung in front of her shoulder, he forced himself to double down on his concentration. Otherwise, he could end up slathering clay on the wrong leg altogether.

And that wouldn't make me look too competent, now would it?

"All set," he said a few moments later, straightening up and patting Baxter on the neck. "Now, all this clay has to do is work its magic overnight."

As Maya raised a less-than-convinced eyebrow, Cal's own eyebrows knitted together. Damn, she was a tough sell, staring him down like he was nothing more than a snake oil salesman.

If this is what I have to look forward to, these two months are going to feel like an eternity.

Cal kept his woeful thoughts to himself, flipping

to a need-to-know question. "So what time should I be here tomorrow? Six a.m.?"

Maya balked slightly. "Um, not if you want to greet me before I have my morning coffee. And trust me, you don't."

Thinking he saw the hint of a smile on Maya's face, Cal readily laughed before realizing he must have imagined amusement on her behalf. Perhaps she needed another cup of that coffee. And *he* could use a strong swig of whiskey right about now, anything to dull his growing impression of a potentially stern taskmaster. Or maybe this was simply Maya's way of making clear who was in charge.

Okay, you're the boss. Can we move forward now?

"During the school year, I usually get here by eight a.m., after my son gets on the school bus," Maya continued. "So, why don't we shoot for that starting time."

The fact that Maya had a child caught Cal by surprise, although he couldn't be sure why. Instinctively, he glanced down at her left hand, noting that there was no wedding ring. Not that this meant anything. Plenty of large-animal vets preferred to have unadorned hands, given that they all too often ended up covered in slop of one kind or another.

"How old is your son?" Cal asked, genuinely curious.

It *seemed* like a harmless enough question, which

was why Maya's suddenly stiffened, guarded body language caught him by surprise.

"He's eight," she replied, after several awkward moments of silence.

Cal smiled and nodded. He knew better than to dig further. Perhaps she had an extreme take on the "keep it professional" motto, a thought that left him more than a tad disappointed. He preferred a casual work environment...a laugh here, a joke there, some chatter about weekend plans...

He sighed inwardly, but adapting to new situations was his forte. It had to be, given that he preferred never staying in one place for too long. So he'd make the best of it, and at least the scenery would be enjoyable. He cleared his throat, only too aware that the colorful Vermont countryside was not the only thing that would be catching his eye for the next couple of months. Although with that frosty attitude...

Cal twisted his mouth to the side. Forget about autumn. Winter had already arrived.

Twenty minutes later, Cal entered the chalet-style cabin that would be his home for the next couple of months. Dropping his truck keys on the kitchen counter, he scanned his surroundings, nodding his head in approval of the rustic vibe.

The silence surrounding him was pierced by a chuckle as an image of Maya slid into his thoughts. She was quite the little spitfire, that was for sure.

Then again, someone of her small stature had to radiate confidence and strength in order to work around horses. They could read these sorts of things. A two-hundred-pound brute of a man emanating fear in their presence? They'd steamroller over him like he was a mere pebble in their path. A one-hundred-pound wisp of a woman who mentally stood her ground? It could turn a snorting, bucking stallion into a docile puppy dog.

All of which begged the question...was he going to be the stallion in this situation?

Don't even go there, mate, he told himself, though he was admittedly intrigued by the prospect. Still, he came here to do a job, and that's what he needed to focus on. Especially since the two-month contract would be over before it had barely begun. But wasn't that his specialty? *Swoop in...and swoop right back out.*

He shook his head, grateful that his interviews had been with Maya's father, Gus, rather than Maya herself. Otherwise, he probably wouldn't have gotten past a coast-to-coast hello via cell phone. She seemed wary of him, and it wasn't a stretch to think that his history of bouncing from one job to the next might have set off her spidey senses. Especially when her own professional background seemed so closely tied to family and the small town of Maplewood.

Cal recalled how Gus had spoken about Maya with so much pride during their interviews, expressing his concern for her well-being as she took on increasingly more responsibilities within the family vet practice. He wondered what it must be like to be part of a tight-knit family, to know they always had your back and you had theirs.

But his brain simply couldn't go there. Then again, how could it? Despite having traveled the world and holding his own in several languages, *family* was one word that held no meaning for him, even in his native English. Not when his mother, a drug-addicted teenager, had disappeared from his life shortly after his birth in Queensland, Australia. But that was still a longer presence than his father, whom he'd never known. And then bouncing around from one foster home to another...

Stop.

Cal's forceful, one-word directive was enough to shake off his chokehold of thoughts. At least for now. But his mind was such that it couldn't be rudderless for long. It had to latch on to something, and as that *something* became an image of Maya, he wondered what her story was. She'd been through a lot—he could see it in her eyes. A reminder that heartache and disappointment spared no one, regardless of the strength of family ties. Perhaps that's why she had her guard up. And though his attraction to her was immediate, he needed to be careful.

Because there was no way he'd want to be another reason for sadness in those soulful light gray eyes.

CHAPTER TWO

THE NEXT MORNING at precisely 8:03 a.m., Maya entered the clinic barn and headed toward Baxter's stall. She was a few feet shy of the gate when Cal popped his head over, prompting her to jump backward.

"Sorry—I didn't mean to scare you," he said.

As sunrays peeked in from the barn windows, illuminating Cal's blue-green eyes, Maya felt her knees tremble. And it wasn't due to her startled hop a few seconds earlier.

"That's okay. I'm used to being the first one here in the morning, and you caught me by surprise—that's all." She cleared her throat, hoping it would also clear her head. "How's he doing?"

Cal flashed a half grin as he held the gate open. "Come see for yourself."

"Wow!" Maya exclaimed moments later as she examined Baxter's pastern area. "I can't believe how much the dermatitis cleared up overnight."

"Lake Mungo scores again," Cal said, prompting a grin from Maya.

She stood up from her kneeling position, not realizing how close she had been squatting next to Cal. Standing just inches away from him now, feeling nearly dwarfed by his six-foot-two, rugged body, Maya felt like the stall walls were closing in on her. How else to explain that she could barely catch her breath?

As Cal's magnetic gaze locked on to hers, she felt like a horse whose fight-or-flight switch had just been triggered. And flight it would be.

Wincing at a jab of pain as she grabbed the stall gate latch with her left arm, Maya nearly stumbled out into the barn aisle, then took a deep breath to calm herself. If she was going to adhere to her "keep it professional" motto, then that also meant not acting like a skittish colt in his presence.

Cal entered the aisle and closed the gate behind him. His eyes were slightly squinted as he cast them in her direction, and something told her it wasn't due to the burgeoning sunlight filtering through the barn.

No, he was sizing her up, trying to discern why she had just acted the way she did. Maya knew there were all sorts of things he could ask or say in this moment—things that would only add to her self-induced uncomfortableness—but to his credit, he merely smiled.

"Well, whatever's next on the agenda, I'll follow your lead," he said.

Maya felt the tightness in her chest begin to recede. "I figured we could go on calls together for the next few days while you get the lay of the land, then after that, we'll divide and conquer. Although, there'll be occasions when we'll need to pair up."

He nodded. "Sounds like a plan."

"Great. Let's check in on our patients here, and then it's off to our first appointment." She paused long enough allow a subdued smile to escape. "I think you'll like where we'll be heading."

Fifteen minutes later, Cal turned to Maya from the passenger seat of her large, fully stocked, capped pickup truck. "Are you going to keep me in suspense?" he asked.

It took several moments for the meaning behind his question to sink in. "Oh—that's right. I said you'd like where we're headed. It's a place called Happy Hooves Horse Rescue."

"A rescue. I like it already," Cal said with a quick but definitive nod.

"I've known Cathy—the owner—since I was a kid. My dad did a lot of pro bono work for the rescue, and it's a tradition I'm more than happy to continue." She turned to Cal, nearly flinching at the way his intense gaze was focused on her with seeming admiration.

"That's great. There are far too many horses in this world that are discarded without a second thought." He paused, clenching his jaw. "That's one of the reasons I left my last gig."

Maya raised an eyebrow. "Oh?"

"I was working at a racetrack in Southern California. Never really gave a huge amount of thought to the horse racing biz, but seeing how so many of the owners cared only about money, and not the welfare of the horses…it was hard to take."

Maya nodded. Cal's concern for the horses had just bumped him up about, oh, one hundred-plus pegs in her eyes.

"Believe me, I know what you mean. In fact, several of the horses at the rescue are young Thoroughbreds that didn't make the cut on the racetrack, and were being shipped to…" Maya stopped, unable to say the word.

As Cal shook his head, eyes blazing, it was clear that she didn't need to.

"Anyway, there are lots of happy endings at Happy Hooves," she said, needing to hear something more positive to focus on, even if it came from her own mouth.

"Happy endings at Happy Hooves. Now that's the kind of happy-happy that I like."

They shared a brief laugh, a much-needed respite from the shared angst over the plight of unwanted equines. Not since George had Maya felt a connection to another vet who seemed to care as deeply as she did about such issues. Even Max, as highly competent as he'd been in veterinary medicine, seemed capable of shutting off the empathy gene whenever it had suited him.

She couldn't shut off that endless well of compassion even if she tried…and something told her the same could be said of Cal.

Ten minutes later, Maya pulled the truck onto the long gravel driveway that wound its way up to the rescue's main buildings.

A tall, slender woman waved from the porch of a white farmhouse, then headed out to meet them.

Dressed in tight jeans, worn cowboy boots and a black T-shirt with white letters that read Horses, Yay!... People, Neigh!, Cathy left no second-guessing as to her priorities in life. Her tanned, weathered face proudly hid none of her sixty-eight years, and the long salt-and-pepper braid that fell halfway down her back only added to her horsewoman mystique.

"Cathy, I'd like you to meet Cal. He's going to be helping out for a bit while my dad starts to transition to retirement."

"Nice to meet you," Cal said as he shook Cathy's hand.

"Same here," Cathy said, eyes squinting as she homed in on him.

Taking a step back, Cathy used her hand as a visor to shield her gaze from the sun, then looked Cal up and down as though she was ready to bid on him at an auction. Little did Maya know that this wasn't so far from the truth.

Cathy stepped slightly to the side, as though sizing up Cal's broad-shouldered physique from another angle.

Maya dropped her head to conceal a muffled snicker. What was next? Opening Cal's mouth and giving his teeth a once-over? Grabbing his leg and flexing it sideways to test his joints? It certainly looked that way.

"Say, how would you like to help out with the horses?" Cathy asked Cal in her no-nonsense, clipped voice. That's how Maya knew Cathy was addressing a human. If she had been talking to one of her horses, her voice would have been much softer.

Cal bent his head to the side, shifting his weight from one leg to the next.

He looked over at Maya, a "what the heck" appeal beaming from his widened eyes. She thought to reassure him with a supportive nod, except that she wasn't quite sure what Cathy was up to, either.

"That's, um, why we're here today—right?" Cal asked as he turned back to Cathy. "To examine and vaccinate some new arrivals?"

Cathy smiled, the creases around her brown eyes deepening. "I'm talking about helping out in another way. We're holding a Hunks for Horses fundraiser in a couple of weeks, and you'd be perfect."

Cal cleared his throat. "Perfect for what?"

"Bringing in the dough."

This time, Maya didn't bother to hide her chuckle. *Damn, this is getting good...*

"Bringing in the..." Cal stopped short of fully repeating Cathy's explanation.

"You just have to strut your stuff on stage, and some lucky gal will be paired up with you for a date," Cathy said matter-of-factly.

Cal ran his fingers through his dark blond hair. "Well, I'm not sure that I've ever been auctioned off on a date before." He turned to Maya, his face softening into a grin. "But if it can help the horses, then I'm game."

"Glad to hear it," Cathy said, pulling her phone out of her back pocket. She stepped back and focused the camera on Cal. "Can you turn your body to the side a bit, and give me some bicep?"

Maya did a double take. She'd heard that Cathy had been briefly married years ago, but since she'd known her, the only males that had caught Cathy's attention were all gelded and trotting on four legs. So to see her size up Cal now like a slab of beefcake was *quite* unexpected. Then again... Maya found it hard to believe that any woman—no matter how dormant her hormones—could be oblivious to Cal's rugged Aussie charms.

Did I just think that?

Maya tried to steer her thoughts in another direction, but her built-in GPS seemed to be set on Cal's muscular arms. She watched with *way* too much enjoyment as Cal posed this way and that, all based on Cathy's eager directives. *Could this get any more surreal?* Maya wondered.

Finally, Cathy appeared to be done, and Maya squelched her impulse to shout out, *Are you sure you don't want another pose?*

"Thanks," Cathy said to Cal. "My niece takes

care of social media updates for the rescue, so I'll be sure to have her plaster your picture everywhere."

Cal was beginning to look uncomfortable again. "I'm not the only bloke signed up for the fundraiser—right?"

"No, but you're the only one everyone will be salivating over," Cathy said, prompting yet another surprised head swirl from Maya. "Trust me. I've got Lonnie, the local sheriff who also plays Santa every year—no costume needed. Let's see, there's also my handyman, Ed. Super nice guy, but has the face of a meerkat. And the body, too, for that matter. And then there's Mike—"

Cal held up his hand and laughed. "That's okay—I think I've heard enough."

Cathy launched into a grin. "Great. Then let's get down to business and go have a look at the new residents."

As Maya and Cal followed Cathy to the nearest paddock, Cal slowed his pace, prompting Maya to do the same.

"You could have warned me that I was walking into a trap," he said, his voice low and eyes flashing with a mix of disbelief and amusement.

"I would've thought this sort of thing was right up your alley," Maya whispered back tersely.

As Cal did a double take, she felt slightly guilty for her harsh reply. *Slightly.*

"I honestly had no idea she was going to ask you to participate in the fundraiser," she quickly added, a half-hearted attempt to neutralize some of the salt she'd thrown into the wound. Which was true. And another truth, one that she was more than happy to keep to herself? There was no way she'd be throwing her name into a hat—or most likely in this case, a stable bucket—and risk the possibility that she'd be the one chosen for a night out on the town with Cal. Not when her top priority was maintaining a strictly professional relationship with him. That's what was clearly best for her...and more importantly, best for Jeremy.

For a split second, she wondered if she was putting the cart before the horse. Why all the inner protests about keeping things professional, when in fact Cal had so far been the perfect gentleman, with not a single inappropriate comment or innuendo tossed her way? Except...if eyes could talk, *his* eyes would be saying *Fancy having some fun on the side while I'm here?* Maybe she was reading a little too much into his stolen glances in her direction, or the physically electrifying vibe that she felt reverberate between them whenever he was near, but there was nothing wrong with being proactive.

Glad we got that resolved, Maya thought triumphantly as she trod onward with determination in her step. Sensing Cal's gaze upon her, she glanced at him sideways, feeling an instant ripple in her resolve. Everything about him was a smorgasbord for the eyes, but this was one buffet she needed to steer clear of.

Maya grimaced. It was never easy turning down dessert, but with a little...okay, a *lot*...of willpower, she could do it.

Cathy led her and Cal into a smaller barn where three new rescues were being temporarily quarantined. It was always a good idea to separate newcomers for at least a few weeks, just to be sure they weren't carrying any contagious diseases that could be transmitted to the rest of the herd.

After Cathy gave a run-through of their backgrounds—an American quarter horse surrendered by his owner due to financial hardship, a Standardbred retired from the racetrack due to a career-ending leg injury and a former Amish-cart-pulling Belgian Draught removed from an auction and spared a potentially life-ending fate—Maya and Cal got down to business.

Working in tandem as they performed thorough physical exams, Maya was almost surprised to find how easy it was to collaborate with Cal. He worked like she did—evaluating physical and behavioral issues based on solid medical guidance, but also through gut instinct. With horses, that instinct often spoke volumes.

All three horses were underweight and in need of a good hoof trim, but once Cathy confirmed the farrier was scheduled for later in the week, and a game plan was agreed upon to safely build up their weight, both Maya and Cal felt it was safe to administer the core vaccines for rabies, tetanus, the mosquito-borne viruses of eastern and western equine encephalitis, and West Nile virus. With mosquito activity at its highest in the fall, Maya felt relieved to know they'd now be protected from these potentially fatal illnesses.

As the trio left the barn and walked back out toward the main buildings, Cal suddenly halted.

"Who's that?" he asked as he nodded toward a caramel-colored horse with a long cream mane in one of several large, fenced pastures. The horse stood by itself, away from a small herd that was contently grazing, its head hanging dejectedly downward.

"That's Molly," Cathy replied. "She's a BLM mustang rounded up two years ago in Nevada. Not sure if you're familiar with the Bureau of Land Management program where they try to place wild horses in homes, but she was bouncing from one adopter to another, and on her way to auction when I intervened and brought her here. I knew what her fate would be if I didn't."

Maya felt a cloud of sadness descend upon her, and as she briefly locked eyes with Cal, she could see that he shared her deep concern with the fate of unwanted horses.

"Do you know why her adopters gave her up?" Cal asked.

"She's withdrawn to the point that she won't assimilate with the herd—never mind bond with a human being. Can't say that I blame her, after she was separated from her family and taken away from the only home she'd ever known."

Cal nodded slightly, his gaze still fixed intently on the mare. "Mind if I go meet her?" he asked, turning back to Cathy, then locking eyes with Maya.

In that moment, there was a knowing exchange between them, a feeling of *we're cut from the same cloth*. She was an American and he an Australian… she'd never left her small-town roots and he apparently couldn't be tied down to any one corner of the globe…yet together they shared a deep empathy and love for horses that transcended words.

"Sure," Cathy said, turning to Maya as Cal strode off toward the pasture. "*Where* did you find that perfect specimen of a man?"

Maya gasped, partly for effect, and partly out of genuine shock that her normally reserved client and friend had just uttered something that seemed miles out of character.

"What?" Cathy retorted with mock defense as she shrugged her shoulders. "I might not have much use for men these days, but that doesn't mean I can't appreciate a good-looking guy who knows a thing or two about horses."

Both women shared a laugh, then looked out onto the field as Cal approached Molly. The mare pricked up her ears, then lifted her head in Cal's direction.

"Well, that's a first," Cathy said in a quiet voice. "Normally, Molly runs off as soon as you approach her."

Maya held her breath as Cal inched his way toward Molly. He had the mare's rapt attention, but Maya wasn't sure how. *Something* was preventing Molly's fight-or-flight instinct to kick in. Was it the energy that Cal emanated, a concept that was pure woo-woo to the average person, but not to someone like herself, who understood how horses could pick up on a person's heartbeat from four feet away? And that was just the beginning of their heightened perceptions.

Maya watched intently as Molly took a step toward Cal. Even from a distance, she could see that the mare was responding to some invisible cue. Whether it was Cal's body language and his energy, or a sixth sense that both human and horse were tapping into, Maya couldn't be sure. But she was mesmerized by what she was witnessing firsthand.

"Amazing," Cathy said in a low voice, her eyes glued to the unexpected scene before her. "Is he a horse vet, or a horse whisperer?"

"It certainly looks like both," Maya said quietly. Which was good news for the horses, but bad news for her. Curtailing her attraction to a man that was based solely on his irresistible looks? That was doable. But when this same man had depth and integrity, and a shared love for and connection to horses...*that* attraction wasn't so easy to outright dismiss. But she'd have to...and she would.

Cal looked up from his deliberate stare at the ground, then cast his eyes—his *soft* eyes—on Molly. If someone was to ask him what the heck "soft eyes" were, he wasn't sure he could adequately explain. It wasn't so much a physical stance as it was a mental and emotional one. It was as if his eyes were verbally saying, *Don't be scared. I won't hurt you.*

When he had first spotted Molly, it was like seeing a ghost. Everything about the mare—from her cream-colored mane and sorrel coat, to her timid and fearful demeanor—reminded him of Flaxxie, the first horse he'd ever bonded with as a young teen. His eyes flickered for a moment before he willed their softness to return, an involuntary response to painful memories dotted amongst happier ones.

It was always a mixed bag of emotions when he looked back on the years that he'd been placed in the care of Thomas and Mabel Crawford, a couple in their late sixties who ran a large horse ranch in the outback. It was the first—and last—time he'd ever felt he was part of a family who cared about him. And it was also here where he quickly developed an affinity for horses that transcended any bond he had ever known.

Flaxxie's mother had tragically died during her

birth, and the young filly had struggled to bond with other mares in the herd, increasingly acting out as they continued to ostracize her. As a fifteen-year-old who'd already experienced a lifetime of disappointment, Cal had found a kindred spirit in Flaxxie. He'd intrinsically understood her angst, the desire to be part of a family, the defiant "Fine, I don't need anyone" attitude in the absence of anyone stepping up to the plate.

So *he* had stepped up, helping to build her confidence on the way to full acceptance within the herd—and with no formal training on his part. But then again, none was needed. He was simply a natural around horses. It was as if he could look into their eyes and see their very soul, sensing their fears or contentment…just as they understood *him* on the deepest level. It was daily equine therapy—before he ever knew that such a healing mode officially existed.

Its effect on him was so powerful that it had spurred his desire to become an equine veterinarian, a lofty goal that he knew would normally be out of reach for someone like himself, without a penny to rub between two fingers. But he had wanted it too much to be deterred. And so he doubled down on his secondary school studies and tagged along on farm visits with the local vet every chance he had. His perseverance had paid off in the form of a full scholarship to a veterinary college in Victoria.

That was one of the happy memories from his time at the ranch.

As Molly snorted, bringing him partially back to the present, Cal wondered if she sensed the darker recollections that tagged along with the happier ones.

Don't go there.

Cal closed his eyes and breathed in deeply, searching for a zen moment to melt away everything but the *now*. Only by being fully present would he be able to connect to Molly. When he opened his eyes again, she tossed her head and pawed at the ground, then took a step closer. She was tentatively in his space now, and it would be easy enough to reach over and gently stroke her face.

But he needed her permission first. Another half step. She was so close now that he could feel her warm breath on his bare forearm. He stood motionless, as though he had all the time in the world. In this moment, everything and everyone else was blocked out. It was just him and Molly…and a silent dance of trust and vulnerability between them.

Several minutes passed, and then Cal spoke quietly. "I'll be back, Molly," he said. Her dark brown eyes seemed to register understanding.

As he approached Maya and Cathy outside of the fence gate a short time later, he couldn't help but notice how they were both viewing him through disbelieving eyes.

"I thought for sure she was going to let you touch

her," Maya said, her long brown ponytail bobbing with every animated word.

"I almost did," Cal said. "But one too-soon move now, and it would be very hard to ever gain her trust." He turned to address Cathy. "I'm not sure if you'd be okay with this, but I'd love to work with Molly during my free time, see if I can bring her out of her shell a bit more."

"'Okay with this'?" Cathy repeated incredulously. "I'd be thrilled! You just established more of a connection with her in five minutes than I've been able to do in almost five months."

Cal smiled. "Great. I really think I can make some significant progress with her. She *wants* to trust—I can just feel it."

"Just be sure she doesn't kick you before the fundraiser," Maya noted with a mischievous twinkle in her eye. "You don't want to be strutting your stuff on stage with a bum knee."

"Good point!" Cathy chimed in as Cal let out a good-natured chuckle.

"Glad you both have my well-being in mind," he said with a wry grin.

After a tour of the rescue, Cal and Maya bid goodbye to Cathy and the horses, then headed for the truck.

Cal felt relieved that the first day of his stint with Equine Associates was rolling out on such a positive note. Any initial qualms he'd had about working with Maya had quickly been nixed. She wasn't the know-it-all, micromanager type that he had worried she might be, questioning his every diagnosis or treatment suggestion. Rather, she seemed to approach horse care much like he did—with an inquisitive mind, a keen eye and a sensitivity to their emotional as well as their physical makeup.

"Mind if I drive?" Cal asked as Maya opened the driver's side door. She was about to hop in, but paused. "No pulling any wheelies."

He laughed. "Promise I won't."

Once they were on the main road, Maya turned to him. "I still can't believe the way you were able to connect with Molly like that. Cathy said she's barely able to get near her—and she's no slouch around horses, obviously. Is it something you were taught, or does it come naturally?"

No one had ever asked him this before, and though Cal knew the answer, it was slow to depart his lips. "Comes naturally, I guess."

"Well, Molly really seemed to gravitate toward you, and it was pretty amazing to watch."

"She reminded me of one of the first horses I ever worked with."

"As a vet?"

"No, it was at a horse ranch in the outback. I was a teenager at the time."

"What was her name?" Maya asked, her voice upbeat.

Perhaps she was expecting some joyful recollections, Cal thought, but nothing could be further from the truth.

His throat clamped shut, rendering any answer impossible. Why did he even bring this up? He'd never mentioned Flaxxie to another person before, in part because of the painful memories that reignited in even a passing reference, but also because they could never understand. But Maya could. She shared his deep compassion for horses, and she wouldn't look at him like he had two heads if he told her things that still haunted him to this day.

Still…he couldn't finish what he started. At least not now. He wasn't ready to be this vulnerable in front of Maya, who he was just getting to know, and maybe he never would.

Stalling for time, Cal stared straight ahead at the road, but he could still feel Maya's eyes upon him as she waited for an answer.

He pressed down slightly on the gas pedal, as though accelerating the truck would drive him out of the dark place where his thoughts had landed. But he was still there, the determined young man in his final year of veterinary school who had lost so much seemingly overnight. When Thomas and Mabel had passed away within months of each other just before his graduation, the ranch that he had called home… and the horses he had deeply cared about…were passed on to their two biological sons, who wanted nothing to do with any of it.

Even now, years later, he could feel the sharp sting

of anger, and the dull pang of helplessness, that had defined his last days in Australia as he tried desperately to ensure that the horses would be cared for. If only he could have bought the ranch himself, but it had been a financial impossibility. He'd done everything in his power—of which he had little at the time—to track down Flaxxie, but he never learned of her fate. His anguish at the time had been debilitating enough to vow to leave the country with his newly acquired degree in hand, a decision he had never regretted.

"Are you okay?" Maya asked, her voice tentative, as though she'd picked up on his sudden shift in demeanor.

Cal forced a smile, scrambling to think of something to say that would instantly lighten the mood. "I'm fine. I was just wondering about what I should wear for my fundraiser debut. I don't know... I'm thinking maybe a pair of backless chaps, minus the jeans?"

He held his breath, hoping that Maya would somehow not notice that he'd evaded her question.

She noticed, he thought as he briefly met her puzzled eyes. But to her credit, she didn't push the matter, and instead let out a throaty chuckle.

"I can't believe you just said that."

Neither could he, considering she was technically his boss, and he had no idea how she'd react to the comment. It was one of those speak first, think later moments...and luckily, it hadn't backfired on him.

It was dusk by the time they pulled into the clinic after their last appointment for the day.

"Looks like my dad's here," Maya said as she glanced at his SUV parked next to the office. "Let's go say hi and let him know I didn't fire you yet."

Cal chuckled. She was kidding, after all...*right*? Still, he breathed a little easier when she turned back to him with a smirk on her face.

"It's the man of the hour!" Gus boomed good-naturedly as they entered the office. "How did your first day on the job go?"

Maya glanced at Cal, her face tired yet beaming. "It went great. Cal here is quite the horse whisperer."

Gus smiled and nodded his approval. "Is that so. Well, can't say that I'm surprised."

Suddenly, the office door opened and a young boy boisterously entered. "Hey, Mom," he said as he headed toward Maya. Cal noticed a flicker of tense surprise on her face, and how she immediately turned back to her dad.

"Oh—I should have mentioned this already," Gus explained, "but Jeremy asked if he could come by with me to visit with the horses." He looked at his grandson. "Everyone A-OK?"

The boy smiled. "Yup. They're eating their hay and farting up a storm."

"Jeremy!" Maya admonished, though she chimed in with a chuckle as Cal burst out laughing.

Gus looked over at Cal. "Jeremy here is a budding horse vet."

Cal smiled. "Runs in the family, I'd say."

His smile faded as he saw a flash of pain on Maya's face. Was it triggered by his comment? He couldn't imagine why. Unless she didn't want her son to become a horse veterinarian…and that certainly didn't make any sense.

"Jeremy, this is Cal," Gus said. "He's going to be working with your mom for the next couple of months."

"Nice to meet you, Jeremy," Cal said, feeling Maya's stern eyes upon him like laser beams set on high as he approached the young boy.

Jeremy looked up at him inquisitively. "You talk funny."

"That's called an accent," Maya said with a hint of amusement in her voice.

"Oh—sorry," Jeremy replied sheepishly. "Where are you from?"

"I'm from Australia," Cal said as he looked down on the freckle-faced boy. "But I've lived pretty much all over the world."

"Wow, that's cool," Jeremy said, prompting low-key laughter from Gus and Maya.

As Cal straightened up, his eye caught a row of framed photos on the side wall. Jeremy followed his gaze, then walked over and pointed to one of the pictures.

"That's me helping my mom examine Crackers."

Cal approached his side and studied the photo of Maya resting the front hoof of what appeared to be a Shetland pony on her bent knee, pointing something out to a younger Jeremy as she did.

"Hmm. Hoof bruise?" Cal asked.

"Stone stuck in the frog. I helped pick it out."

"Way to go!" Cal said, genuinely impressed that he was honing future veterinary skills at such a young age.

Another photo caught his attention, this one of a younger Gus standing proudly with one arm around the shoulder of a school-age Maya, a large vet bag dangling from his other arm. The top of Maya's head barely reached Gus's chest, but even so, her smiling face exuded the same determination and grit that he saw in her now.

Cal's lips silently curved upward as he focused in on a small vet bag in her grip. It was even embroidered with fancy cursive writing that read Maya's Vet Kit. He wondered if it had been a Christmas or birthday gift. *No Barbie dolls for you, right?*

"That's me and my dad," Jeremy said, pointing to another photo. In it, Maya stood with her arm around the waist of an outdoorsy-looking man, who held a toddler-aged Jeremy up against his chest with one arm. Given that he wore a Northern Vermont Equine Associates T-shirt like Maya did in the photo, he must have been a fellow vet, Cal reasoned.

If they were divorced, was he still in the picture? He certainly didn't look like the type to run out on his family. Cal frowned at his thoughts. As if he could tell *anything* about the man by merely glancing at a single celluloid moment from the past.

Feeling eyes upon him, he turned to find Maya watching him intently, and as a quiet stillness descended over the room, he wondered where all the oxygen had gone.

Glancing at his watch without actually reading the numbers, he declared, "Well, I think I'll go check up on our patients in the barn before dark."

Closing the office door behind him as he stepped outside, Cal looked up at the purplish-orange sky, drawing in a deep breath. It had been quite the day. And working with Maya could only mean one thing…it was going to be quite the two months.

CHAPTER THREE

MAYA GRIPPED THE steering wheel of her personal SUV as she drove from her house to the clinic. It was Saturday morning—technically a day off—but that never stopped her from swinging by the main barn for a quick check on onsite patients.

All around her, the colorful brilliance of a Vermont autumn was in high gear. Quite simply, she didn't believe there could possibly be a more beautiful place—or time of year—on the planet, and the seasonal influx of leaf-peeping tourists seemed to second this notion.

Yet, despite the scenes of splendor that whizzed by the side windows, Maya was feeling distracted and tense. An image of Cal flashed in her mind, as if to say, *Am I the reason you can't focus right now?* Maya twisted her mouth to the side, refusing to inwardly reply. *As if I don't know the answer to that question...*

Cal's first week on the job had officially wrapped up yesterday, and Maya couldn't imagine a more competent colleague. He didn't just know his way around horses...he knew a way into their souls. And that, in her experience, was an incredible gift.

Still, there was no shortage of caution lights flickering around him. He jumped from one job to the next, and in just a couple of months, he'd be departing this current one as well. He seemed to be running from *something*, that was for sure. From boredom? Adult responsibilities? A jilted ex-lover?

Maya snorted at this last improbable possibility. Or maybe it wasn't so improbable, given that she of the "I can't be bothered to look" missive had in fact been looking. A lot.

Not that this was Cal's fault, of course. He couldn't help the fact that he was quite literally a Hunk for Horses. That had been apparent from the moment they had first met. But his deep caring and compassion for equines—something that had exposed a vulnerability behind his *very* solid exterior? That had come as more of a surprise.

And now, as Maya replayed in her mind all the instances when she'd treated him dismissively since they had first met, she was feeling pangs of regret. He'd been nothing but friendly toward her and her dad and Jeremy. Maybe it was time to cut him some slack.

As she pulled into the clinic's long driveway, Maya vowed to make amends when the time and circumstances were right. She wouldn't address her behavior to Cal directly, but perhaps she could offer a goodwill gesture of some sort when the opportunity arose.

Yes, I can do that...

Maya's thoughts were cut short as she spotted

Cal's dark blue truck in one of the parking spots by the main barn.

Forehead creased as questions swirled in her mind, Maya quickly exited her truck and headed for the barn entrance.

"Morning!" Cal exclaimed as he walked out from the barn into the sunlit morning. "I thought I heard a car pull up."

"It's Saturday," Maya said as she viewed him quizzically. "Your day off."

Cal flashed a one-sided grin. "Yours too—isn't it?"

Maya wasn't sure how to respond to that observation. "I'm part owner of the practice. I never have a day off," she finally said, only half kidding.

"Well, that's no fun." There was a twinkle in Cal's eye that was *fun* personified.

Maya pretended to herself that she hadn't noticed this.

"I came by to check on Razzle," Cal explained, referring to the American paint horse gelding that was being rehabbed for a torn suspensory ligament in his hind leg.

He came by on his day off to check on one of the horses! Maya held her breath as she let that thought sink in.

"I came by to check on him, too. How's he doing?"

"He seems fine. Must have tweaked something yesterday, but whatever it was, it's gone now. Mark said he saw no new signs of lameness this morning."

Maya breathed a sigh of relief. "That's great news."

She knew that Mark, a fourth-year veterinary student who worked on weekends as a vet tech at the clinic, would have caught anything that was amiss. Still, she remembered her own days as a final-year student on the brink of becoming a bona fide veterinarian. You could never have too many highly trained eyes weighing in on cases while trying to rack up actual field experience.

"Anything you'd like me to do while I'm here?" Cal asked.

"No, but thanks for asking. Go enjoy your day off."

Cal smiled and nodded, seeming to hesitate slightly before turning to head to his truck.

Maya watched as he started to walk away, then allowed impulse to take over. "Have you ever had pancakes and maple syrup before?" she quickly blurted out, before she had a chance to change her mind about following through with her goodwill gesture.

Cal turned and looked at her quizzically, as though wondering if this was a trick question. "Sure."

"No—I mean *real* maple syrup."

"If you mean something other than artificial syrup with fake maple coloring and a lot of fine print that says Bad for Your Health...then the answer is no."

Maya snickered. "Come on," she said, nodding toward her SUV.

Cal looked equal parts confused and intrigued. "Where are we going?"

"Marie's Breakfast Nook in downtown Maplewood. It has the best melt-in-your-mouth pancakes and *pure* Vermont maple syrup."

"Maplewood has a downtown?" he asked cheekily.

"Ha! Yes, but no one would mistake it for a metropolis, I can tell you that."

Cal grinned. "All the better."

The breakfast café was bustling with local regulars and tourists when Maya and Cal entered after a short drive over. With wooden furniture, gingham place settings and the scintillating aroma of freshly baked muffins and cinnamon rolls, the café was a feast for the senses.

"There's a spot," Maya said as she pointed to a booth tucked away in the far-left corner that had just been vacated by another couple. "Let's grab it fast!"

They were barely seated before a young waitress whizzed by, then paused and backtracked.

"Coffee?" she asked in a chirpy voice as she cleared the plates with one hand and deftly cleaned the tabletop with a damp cloth pulled from her apron pocket.

"Sure," Maya replied.

"Please," Cal said with a friendly nod.

"How many cups today will that be?" Cal asked with a grin once the waitress departed.

"Maybe my third—but who's counting?"

Cal chuckled as he scanned the laminated one-page menu. "Pumpkin pancakes," he said with curiosity as he perused the menu.

"Oh—you've got to try those," Maya said enthusiastically. "They are *delicious*."

As Maya scanned her own menu, she suddenly became aware of a deafening silence. Just moments earlier, she could barely hear herself think above the din of overlapping conversations around them...and now this?

She peered up at Cal, who also seemed keenly aware that something was amiss. "Did it just suddenly get quiet in here?" he asked in a near whisper.

Maya discreetly nodded, then scanned the room. Given that they were quite literally in their own little corner, she didn't think they could possibly have drawn the attention of others. But either she was being totally paranoid...or every patron was in fact looking their way. Actually, that wasn't quite accurate. Every *female* customer was pointedly staring in their direction.

"Do I have something on my face?" she whispered to Cal as she leaned in closer for some privacy. At least what little they had under the circumstances.

Cal's eyes darted around him. "Just the same look of surprise that I have." Suddenly, his lightly tanned face turned ghostly white. "Oh, no. No, no, no..."

"What?" Maya exclaimed in a hoarse whisper, her heart now racing. She grabbed his forearm, then pulled her hand back as though she had touched a burning stove.

"Sorry," she said of her grab-now-think-later reaction, though in that split second of feeling the warmth of his skin on the palm of her hand, her true feeling could best be summed up as: *Sorry, NOT sorry!*

Cal glanced down to where she'd touched his arm, his eyes lingering there several moments before looking back up at her. Locked into a mutual gaze, she felt the magnetic pull of attraction dance between them. Only when she forced herself to avert her eyes away—*we're just colleagues, after all*—did Cal nod to a tent-shaped advertising display that was propped up in the middle of the table. She stared at it for several moments, then slapped her hand over her mouth to muzzle her laughter.

"Not funny," Cal said in a low growl, though there was no mistaking the reluctant smirk on his face.

Maya picked up the display and discreetly read the print aloud. "'Don't miss our Hunks for Horses fundraiser on September 20 at the Maplewood Grange. Throw your name into the bucket for the chance to win a date with one of these dreamy, horse-loving hunks! Tickets are fifty dollars each—no limit to the number of purchases. All proceeds will benefit the Happy Hooves Horse Rescue.'"

Cal squeezed his eyes shut. "I'm afraid to look around, but they're probably on every table—am I right?"

"Ah...yup," Maya confirmed. "And right now, every woman in here is looking at you and licking her lips."

Maya knew that Cal assumed she was exaggerating in order to needle him further...except that she wasn't. Not that she could blame all the rapt gazes in his direction.

Cal sunk further into his chair. "I think I want to disappear."

"Oh, come now. It's for the horses—just keep remembering that." Maya paused, shaking her head in astonishment. "Although, I have to say—I've always thought of Cathy as a salt-of-the-earth horsewoman with little patience for the business end of things. But turns out she definitely has a bit of a shrewd marketer in her!" Maya held up the display. "I mean—look at this!"

Cal sighed, cupping the side of his head with his hand. "Believe me, I can't unsee it if I tried."

Maya chuckled as she continued to study the advert. To say that Cal's photo was the most prominently displayed was an understatement. His bicep-baring pose was encased in a large circle that was front and center, with smaller circles surrounding him that contained pictures of the other men. The only thing missing was a string of blinking neon lights around his photo. Maya had no doubt that if such an adornment had been an option, Cathy would have personally slapped it on every display.

"Looks like you'll be the main course at Hunks for Horses," she teased.

"Poor Ed," Cal said as he allowed himself a quick glimpse of the photos. "He really *does* look like a meerkat."

Maya laughed, then gave a brief shrug of her shoulders. "That's okay. Meerkats are cute."

Cal's focus swiftly reverted back to Maya. "Does that mean you'll be rooting for a date with him instead of me at the fundraiser?"

Cal's brash question, coupled with an even brasher smile, left Maya sitting on the hot seat. Whether it was actually the seat that was hot, or herself, didn't matter. She needed to redirect the conversation—and fast.

"Here you go," the waitress said as she appeared at the table with a coffeepot in hand. Maya was used to caffeine coming to the rescue, but not quite like it did in this instance.

"Cheers," she said as she raised her mug to Cal's.

He toasted her back, either oblivious to her deliberate segue, or gallant enough to pretend otherwise.

"So, what do you think so far of Maplewood?" she asked, further cementing a change of subject.

"I can see why you like living here. You've got mountains, four beautiful seasons and so far the people seem very friendly. Maybe not as much as the horses—but close."

Maya sputtered on a sip of coffee. "Oh, that's too funny. Well, we New Englanders do have a reputation of being a bit, shall we say, reserved with our friendliness. But I tend to think of it as kind of like the difference between dogs and cats."

Cal raised an amused eyebrow. "I *think* I know where you're going with this, but humor me anyway."

"Dogs like everyone, but cats—you have to earn their like. That's how it is with a lot of New Englanders. Or so they say…"

Cal leaned back in his chair, a devilish smile on his face. "So have I earned your like yet?"

This time, Maya choked on her coffee. Was he really going to go there? Still, as she caught a mischievous twinkle in his eye, it was clear he was keeping it lighthearted, so she decided to do the same. "I don't *dis*like you, so that's a start."

"Meow."

Maya laughed again. He certainly had a way of removing any *dis* from *dislike*.

"So, have you lived here your whole life?"

Maya nodded. "I have, except during my college years in upstate New York. It's beautiful up there, too, but this has always been home to me."

"What about siblings? Any brothers or sisters?"

"I'm an only child, believe it or not." Seeing the look of surprise on Cal's face, she added, "My parents wanted to have more kids, but it wasn't in the cards. I guess that's another reason why I've stayed in the area. When my mom passed away several years ago, it was incredibly hard on my dad—as

I'm sure you can imagine. Jeremy and myself are all he has left."

In the crosshairs of Cal's intense gaze, Maya felt like he was sizing her up...and very much liking how the pieces fit together. "Your dad's lucky to have a daughter like you."

Maya smiled, both appreciative of the compliment and slightly uncomfortable being under a prolonged spotlight.

Time to flip the conversation around.

"So what about you? You said it yourself last night—that you've lived all over the world. Do you have a favorite place?"

"I haven't been *everywhere*, mind you," Cal said, looking upward as though conducting a quick inventory of previous residences.

"Yet," Maya replied with a wry grin.

"Let's see... Switzerland was pretty amazing."

"That doesn't surprise me," Maya said, instantly conjuring up images of alpine meadows strewn with wildflowers. "But do they have pure maple syrup made from local trees?"

Cal chuckled. "Not sure about that, to be honest. I only know about the watches and cheese."

Maya smirked. "What about Australia? Do you ever miss it? I imagine you must still have family there."

Cal's smile faded faster than Maya could say the words *wrong question* in her mind. But *why* was it wrong? It seemed like an innocuous-enough inquiry. Unless, of course, he in fact was harboring some dark secret from his past. She certainly hoped that wasn't the case.

"Are you ready to order?" the waitress asked as she suddenly appeared at the table.

Saved by the pancakes, Maya thought as Cal wasted no time relaying his order of pancakes, hash browns and orange juice to the waitress. He probably would have ordered fried rubber if it meant a chance to change the subject—or so it seemed.

When the conversation resumed a short time later, Maya made sure to skirt any potentially triggering subject matter.

So, nothing about my past or his. Maybe talk about the weather?

"I do love the cool autumn air," Cal said, unknowingly on cue.

Maya managed a half smile. "Remember that when 'cool' transitions to 'frigid.'"

Cal appeared nonplussed. "I had a four-month gig in Alaska at the height of winter a few years ago, so I'm prepared."

Maya struggled to maintain a smile in the midst of Cal's revelation. It should have been something that made her chuckle, but instead, she was filled with unease. Why did he feel the need to hop from one job—and hence, one place—to another? Was it truly a matter of benign wanderlust, or was there more to it than that?

She pushed her concerns aside for the sake of a peaceful outing.

"Can I get you anything else?" the waitress asked once they had finished their meals, approaching their table with a check in hand.

"We're all set, thanks," Maya said, opening her purse to grab her bank card.

"I've got this," Cal said as he reached for his wallet.

Maya held out her hand in the waitress's direction. "No, let me—"

"Actually," the waitress interjected. "The bill's been paid."

Maya and Cal exchanged surprised glances.

"By who?" Maya asked.

The waitress sported a conspiratorial grin as she pointed at a table toward the center of the café. Maya's eyes widened as a trio of young, attractive women waved in their direction. As one stood up, tossing her long honey-blond hair off her shoulders before making her way over, Maya felt her throat clamp shut.

"Uh-oh…" Cal said quietly under his breath. "Is it too late to hide under the table?"

Given that the woman was clearly a looker, Maya was secretly pleased by Cal's less-than-enthused observation.

Like a heat-seeking missile, Cal's admirer quickened her step as she closed in on the table, her eyes laser-focused on the prize. The only thing missing was a big red bow on Cal's head.

"Hi there," she said to him, conveniently ignoring Maya as though she were merely an added condiment at the table. "I'm Susie."

Cal smiled, quickly glancing at Maya before shaking the slender, manicured hand before him. "Cal. Nice to meet you."

Susie's fake eyelashes fluttered like writhing centipedes around her widened eyes. "Oh, wow! Are you Australian? It doesn't say that in your write-up."

Cal looked about as comfortable as if he were sitting on a pincushion—minus the cushion. "I guess they were trying to keep the focus on the horses," he said with the slightest hint of impatience in his voice. But given that it was paired with a polite smile, his borderline annoyance seemed to sail over Susie's well-coiffed head.

"Oh, you're too funny," Susie said, reaching over to brush her hand over his forearm.

Maya's eyeballs popped out so hard that she half expected to hear them bounce off the tabletop.

Unfortunately, Susie wasn't quite finished. "Well, I came over here to let you know my friends and I are in town from New Jersey for another week—just in time to attend the fundraiser. In fact, we've already bought our tickets."

"That's great," Cal said with restrained enthusiasm. "Happy Hooves Horse Rescue will put the donations to good use."

Susie bent down to whisper in his ear. "I bought five tickets—which means five chances that I'll win a date with you."

Having honed her hearing to be almost on par with that of horses, Maya caught every overly inflected word.

Suddenly, Susie turned to her with narrowed raccoon eyes. In that moment, all Maya could think was how much she loved raccoons—as she did all critters—and that Susie should apologize to them for species misappropriation.

But before Maya had a chance to even silently react, Susie turned her attention back to Cal. "Um, you're single—right?"

Maya watched as Cal's Adam's apple rose and fell like a weighted ball in his throat. "I am," he replied...tersely? Sheepishly? Perhaps another adverb? Maya struggled to read into the tone of his response, but then quickly caught herself.

It doesn't matter... He's a temporary colleague who joined me for breakfast—end of story!

Which meant Susie could flirt all she wanted with Cal...and vice versa.

Not surprisingly, Susie seemed pleased with Cal's relationship status. "I just wanted to be sure the rescue isn't setting up a date with someone's husband, you know?" She play-slapped Cal's arm, then tossed her hair back over shoulder. "I'm silly like that."

Maya half rolled her eyes, straightening them out

just in time to catch Cal's amused look in her direction.

Ten minutes later, Maya and Cal headed down the sidewalk to Maya's SUV.

"Are you sure you don't want be my fundraiser date and save me from that barracuda?" he asked.

"I don't know...she seems like your type," Maya deadpanned.

"*Pffftt!* Yeah...*no*."

Maya chuckled, perhaps enjoying his heated denial a little too much. "Your date will be the luck of the draw—remember? That's how these things work. Cathy will dip her hand into the bucket and pull out a name. It might be Susie, given that she's stacked the odds, or it might not."

"Hopefully not," Cal said between slightly clenched teeth.

"Besides, it's never a good thing for colleagues to cross that line."

Cal glanced at her sideways as they continued walking in sync. "What line are we talking about?"

Maya wasn't buying his feigned ignorance. "You know what I mean."

"We just had breakfast together. What's the harm in dinner—especially one that's for a good cause like Happy Hooves?" He paused just long enough for a subdued grin to cross his lips. "Or is it only meals with Vermont maple syrup that are allowed?"

Maya cast him an "okay, wise guy" look. "Just trust me on this." There was *so* much more she could say on the matter...but she also knew it was best to steer clear from anything too personal. Not that Cal, he of the "can't talk about my homeland" mantra, should have a problem with that, she thought pointedly.

Cal sighed inwardly as they turned a corner and continued walking toward the side street where Maya's SUV was parked. It wasn't that he didn't understand the obvious, which was that his fundraiser date would be determined by an anonymous piece of paper pulled out of a bucket. But boy, Maya had *really* jumped on the opportunity to squelch any possibility of them ever straying from a strictly-colleagues stance. Still, he wasn't about to let the matter drop altogether, if for no other reason than she looked so cute when she was annoyed.

"Well," he began as nonchalantly as possible, "since I have to pick the restaurant for my fundraiser date, can you at least suggest a few good ones in the area?" Silence. Followed by more silence. Cal cocked his head to the side in Maya's direction. "That wasn't a trick question, by the way."

She looked up at him. "I'm just trying to think of a place. There are a couple of nicer restaurants that come to mind, but one closed a year ago, and the other is under new ownership, so I can't vouch for how good it is now."

Cal sighed for effect. "Geez, you're not making this easy. Don't worry—I'm not asking you out," he said, wondering if he sounded as unconvincing on this declaration as he felt. "Just looking for some restaurant recommendations. I mean, where did you go on your last date? I'm assuming not McDonald's."

Maya shot him a perturbed glance. "I haven't been on a date in a while. By choice," she added curtly. "I don't have time for that sort of thing right now."

Something about the sharpness behind Maya's reply told Cal that time wasn't the only thing holding her back from stepping out with a male companion. Still, he'd already witnessed enough to know that between a grueling clinic schedule and raising Jeremy as a single parent, she was doing her best to keep a number of plates spinning in the air. If anyone deserved a night to be wined and dined in an upscale venue, no work beeper or chore list in sight, it was Maya. And the fact that he'd be able to spend more one-on-one time with her without a pitchfork or a muddy pasture in sight? Well, that was just a bonus. Correction—a *huge* bonus.

All of which meant…if she wasn't going to agree to such a night out on the town willingly, then he'd need to find a more underhanded way to make it happen. But how?

Your date will be the luck of the draw—remember?

As Maya's earlier forceful reminder popped back into his thoughts, Cal nodded to himself and smiled.

"What's so funny?" she asked as she side-eyed him suspiciously.

He shrugged, his smile widening even more. "Nothing. Nothing at all."

Maya was glad that Cal had dropped the subject of dating on the drive back to the clinic. She still couldn't figure out whether he genuinely wanted to go on a date with her, fundraiser or otherwise, or if he'd been rattling her cage just to provoke a reaction. *I guess I gave him one*, she thought, wishing she could have more of a poker face—and attitude.

Truth was, his flirtatious manner left her feeling both elated and cautious. Elated because it indicated that her attraction to him was not one-sided. And cautious because she knew she had to maintain a strictly professional relationship. And while she trusted herself to do the right thing, that didn't mean it would be easy.

As she pulled into the clinic parking area, Maya was surprised to see her dad and Jeremy lingering outside the barn.

"It's my two favorite guys," she said as she headed over, with Cal close behind. "Is everything okay?"

"Everything's fine," Gus said with a smile. He turned to his grandson. "Jeremy here called me this morning to say he was bored and wanted to come see the horses."

"Jeremy!" Maya exclaimed with mock indignation, hand on her hip. "I asked if you wanted to come to the barn with me this morning, and you said no."

"I was still watching cartoons," he said matter-of-factly, eliciting all-around laughter.

"Say," Gus began, "I'm thinking of taking a ride to Carlisle Orchard to do some apple picking. Would you two like to join us?"

Maya couldn't help but notice how Jeremy looked at Cal, and not her, with almost visibly bated breath as he awaited an answer.

Cal seemed to realize this as well, glancing at Maya before replying to Gus. "Actually, I called Cathy earlier this morning to see if I could come by to work with Molly, so I'll be heading over there soon. But apple picking sounds fun. Maybe another time?"

Jeremy's face instantly lit up. "Can I go with you?" he asked eagerly, looking to Cal and then Maya.

"Honey, I'm sure Cal needs to focus one-on-one with Molly," Maya explained, doing her best to downplay her apprehension.

As Cal looked in her direction, she sensed he disagreed with her assumption, but was hesitant to step into a parental quagmire.

Maya's shoulders dropped. Was she making the right call for Jeremy? That's what mattered most in this moment. He had met Molly on more than one occasion, and each time had been clearly drawn to the timid mustang. Her fear-based, skittish behavior made her too unpredictable for Maya to allow Jeremy to ever have closer proximity than that afforded by a sturdy fence between them, but it hadn't dampened his fascination with her.

"You don't want me to go?" Jeremy asked Cal directly.

"It's fine with me," Cal said carefully. "But if your mum's not comfortable with the idea…"

"I'm sure Jeremy knows to give Cal space while he's working with Molly," Gus offered, turning to his grandson and adding, "Right?"

Jeremy nodded. "I won't get close—I'll just watch." He turned to Maya. "Please?"

Maya bit her bottom lip, feeling three sets of eyes staring at her intently.

Perhaps she needed to rethink her stance. Yes, she was trying to protect Jeremy from a repeat of what had happened with Max. But he was older now. And surely he knew that Cal was strictly her colleague, not also her boyfriend, as was the case with Max.

Plus, there was no possibility that this was going to change. Right?

I said, right?

Maya swallowed hard. Of course that was right. It wouldn't be long before Cal was on to his next chapter in life. Or, maybe it was more like his next few pages. To complete a chapter, you had to actually commit to something. And that didn't seem to be part of his playbook.

"Mom?" Jeremy asked, snapping Maya out of her thoughts. "Can I go?"

Maya bunched her lips together as she looked

at her son. He wanted this so badly, and it wasn't fair to deny him the opportunity to see a real horse whisperer in action.

Let go of the other stuff, she told herself.

"You can come, too," Cal said, sounding as though he hoped she would.

"I have a Maplewood Community Events Committee volunteer meeting at noon, so I won't be able to go. I can't miss planning for the October Harvest Fair, now can I?" She paused to grin, but also to push through her fears. "But you can go, Jeremy. Just make sure you listen to Cal. He's going to need some space and quiet to work with Molly, but you'll learn a lot just from watching him. I know I did the other day."

As Maya locked eyes with Cal, she could almost physically feel his appreciation—not to mention surprise—at her comment.

"Well, looks like I'll be picking apples by myself," Gus said with a one-sided grin.

"Do you want to come with us?" Cal asked.

"Appreciate the offer, but I'm craving a good McIntosh apple. Plus, if I know Cathy, she'll stick a pitchfork in my hand and put me to work instead."

Cal laughed, as did Maya. But as Cal and Jeremy drove off a short time later, she turned to her dad with angst in her eyes.

He hugged her shoulders from the side. "Relax, Maya. This will be good for Jeremy." When she didn't immediately respond, he hugged her even tighter. "I know what you're thinking."

"Do you?" she snapped, before shaking her head. "I'm sorry."

"Don't be. I understand. You don't want Jeremy getting too attached to Cal, but he's older now and I think he's looking at this as a chance to learn more about natural horsemanship. That's all."

Maya looked up at her dad and smiled. His eyes, both kind and wise, instantly helped blunt the edge of her worries.

"Besides," he added, "it'll be good for Jeremy to be around a strong male figure, someone he can aspire to."

Maya was about to point out that emulating someone who seemed incapable of putting down roots *anywhere* was probably not the best role model. But she knew what her dad meant. Jeremy loved horses, and had already talked about following in the family footsteps toward a career in equine medicine. If George were still here, he'd be that perfect male role model.

We'll skip over Max. But George wasn't here. And Cal *was*.

"You okay?" Gus asked, pulling Maya back to the present.

Maya looked up at him and smiled. "Yes," she replied, hoping she wouldn't live to regret her answer.

CHAPTER FOUR

CAL WAS A few minutes into the drive to Happy Hooves Horse Rescue when he glanced over at Jeremy, and it suddenly hit him: This was the first time as an adult that he could recall spending one-on-one time with someone who *wasn't* an adult.

He let that thought sink in, realizing how crazy it sounded—even to himself. It wasn't that he didn't like kids. Quite the opposite, actually. But the opportunity to spend some quality time with a child or even a young teen had never really presented itself. And the reason was quite simple. One had to have family in order to play the role of uncle or older cousin or brother.

He thought of previous romantic relationships, several of which he'd considered serious at the time…albeit serious by his "let's enjoy each other's company exclusively…while I'm here" standards. A couple of those women had young children, but even so, he hadn't been fully enough entwined in their lives to merit one-on-one outings.

Glancing to the side at Jeremy, he wondered what it would be like if he'd gotten a different start in life. Would he be settled down somewhere with a family of his own? He'd still be a horse vet—that was nonnegotiable. But would he be looking over to the passenger seat now at his own son or daughter? Would they share his love of horses, and perhaps be joining him for a horse sanctuary visit—just like Jeremy was now? Would their mother be like Maya—

Whoa!

Cal suddenly hit the brakes, as though trying to dodge a thought that was both disconcerting and unexpected. He'd never before even entertained the idea of having a family of his own, and yet suddenly, the notion had seeped into his psyche. *Could it be because—*

Cal cut off his own question, but not before an image of Maya flashed in his mind, perhaps providing an answer regardless.

"Sorry about that," he said, turning to Jeremy to make sure everything was okay.

"Was something in the road?"

"Yeah…it was, um, a squirrel, I think. But it ran off in time."

Even though the squirrel was fictional, Cal couldn't in good conscience suggest anything less than a safe getaway.

"Good," Jeremy said, looking back with eyes that were nearly translucent gray. *Just like Maya's.* Seeing those eyes made Cal feel as though Maya's essence was somehow in the truck with them. He found himself wishing that she was there in person, and swallowed hard as this revelation reverberated through him.

Pulling into the Happy Hooves parking area fifteen minutes later, Cal was grateful for the chance to hyperfocus on Molly. At the very least, it would keep his thoughts from wandering into off-limits territory.

"I see you brought a helper along," Cathy said as the trio convened in the aisle of the main barn. With a wink, she reached over and tousled Jeremy's hair. At least she didn't slap him on the rump like a prized yearling, Cal thought.

"He wants to learn the way of the force," Cal replied with a wink of his own.

"Lucky you," Cathy said to Jeremy. "You're learning from an equine Jedi Master."

Jeremy looked up at Cal and smiled. "Is Molly outside?" he asked, turning back to Cathy.

"She's in a smaller pasture today by herself. She finally made an attempt to approach the herd the other day, and Moxie and Storm bullied her away."

Cal's smile flattened out. He knew it was just normal horse behavior, an alpha mare and gelding asserting their top of the pecking order. Still, he wished Molly's first attempt at assimilation had gone smoother.

Looking down at Jeremy, he said, "Why don't you head out and say hi to Molly. But don't go inside the pasture," he added, having been given his marching orders on that subject by Maya earlier as he'd been getting ready to leave. "I'll be out in just a minute."

As Jeremy eagerly headed off, Cal turned to Cathy. "Say, Cathy, I wanted to ask you something."

She raised an eyebrow. "No, you can't back out of the Hunks for Horses fundraiser. Ticket sales are soaring, and we've had more than a few inquiries asking if you're actually just an AI-generated image created to boost sales."

Cal chuckled and shook his head. "So that's what the world's coming to. Nice."

Cathy grinned. "You have to understand—all the townsfolk know the other men who are being raffled off. They've never seen you before, and let's just say your picture's got some people champing at the bit."

Cal smirked at the horse analogy, but his amusement was short-lived as Cathy expounded further.

"In fact, there's one gal who's called here a few times offering a nice chunk of change if I rig the winner in her favor."

"Don't tell me her name is Susie."

Cathy cocked her head to the side. "As a matter fact, it is. Do you know her?"

"I ran into her at..." Cal paused, deciding the less that was said, the better. "Never mind. Let's just say she's the persistent type."

"I did get that," Cathy replied, her amused eyes reading his uncomfortable body language. Damn, it was hard to hide something from a horse person, he thought.

"Anyway—what were you going to ask me?"

Cal took a deep breath. *C'mon, buckaroo. You*

had this all worked out in your head just a few hours ago—remember? You can do this.

He cleared his throat. "I was wondering if you'd be able to, uh…"

"Spit it out, boy!"

Cal jumped slightly in place, half expecting Cathy to pull a crop out from behind her back. It was now or never. "Okay, if I donate five hundred dollars to the rescue, would you make it so that Maya is the one who's drawn as my date?"

Cathy appeared momentarily frozen as Cal's question sank in. "Well, I'll be damned. You're trying to bribe me."

Cal's eyes bulged. "No—no, it's not like that! I was planning to donate the five hundred dollars regardless. But I just thought… I mean, it would be nice to take Maya out for a night on the town, that's all. I can see how hard she works, and after her injuries and all…"

Okay, I'll be quiet now, Cal thought as he pondered how far he'd plunged in Cathy's eyes.

She studied him closely for several moments. "You could just ask her out on a date, you know."

Cal sighed, his shoulders dropping. "Actually, I can't. Maya's made it clear that she has no interest in dating anyone, especially a colleague. Or maybe it's just me."

Cathy looked Cal up and down in a way that made him momentarily question whether he remembered to put on clothes. "Nah—it's not you."

"That's good," he replied, not sure what else he could say in the moment.

Cathy bunched her lips together and nodded. "I guess I shouldn't be surprised. She got burned badly by another vet in the practice."

"Oh...?" Cal knew it was none of his business, but the one-word comment still slipped out.

Cathy paused. "I probably shouldn't say anymore, since it's not my story to tell."

Cal pursed his lips together as he silently sucked in a breath. Of course. It *wasn't* any of his business, really. Well...maybe a *little*, given that whatever had happened with the other vet seemed to have deterred her from dating anyone—especially a colleague.

But as Jeremy raced back into the barn, a look of near terror in his eyes, that thought would have to wait.

"Something's wrong with Molly," he said breathlessly. "She's walking weird, and her head is like... it's stuck sideways."

The words hit Cal like a nail-spiked thunderbolt. This was not good. Not good at all.

He froze for all of a second, then ran out of the barn, with Cathy and Jeremy initially on his heels, until he quickly accelerated well beyond them.

"Whoa, girl," he said as he reached Molly, grabbing her halter to help steady her. To his gut-wrenching dismay, Jeremy hadn't been exaggerating. Molly looked at him through fearful eyes...but the fear was different this time. It was as if she knew that something was wrong with her body. He winced at her head tilt, so uncomfortable to even view, and he felt her muscle under his hand as he brushed it across her neck.

"I need a lead rope!" he called back, not taking his eyes off Molly as he did.

"Here!" Jeremy exclaimed a minute later, handing a rope to Cal. "Cathy called my mom."

"Good," Cal said as calmly as possible, hoping to stem any further fear or alarm on behalf of Jeremy. He'd intended for Cathy to enter the pasture with a rope and not Jeremy, but it was too late to change that now. "Why don't you go in front of me, just to be safe."

He snapped the hook onto Molly's halter, waiting for Jeremy to clear the area before slowly walking backward, gently coaxing Molly to follow. Her gait was both hesitant and shaky, like a drunk sailor trying to find his way back to the ship. Whatever was going on with Molly was neurological—of that, he was certain.

Still focusing his highly trained eyes on even the slightest movements or behavior that could provide diagnostic clues, Cal ran the possible scenarios through his mind. Mosquito-borne illnesses and rabies were the most obvious culprits, but he couldn't imagine Molly hadn't been vaccinated in the spring, as was typical. He'd confirm this with Cathy, but in the meantime, he wondered if Molly could have a head injury, although in the absence of other horses nearby, that seemed unlikely. Unless she'd been kicked earlier when she was out with the herd—another question he'd need to run by Cathy.

All of which left equine protozoal myeloencephalitis—or EPM, as it was most commonly known—high on the list of possibilities. Cal drew in a deep breath. At least EPM was not an absolute death sentence, unlike rabies and 90 percent of EEE cases. A parasitic disease most commonly transmitted when a horse came into contact with opossum feces, EPM was survivable when caught early and treated aggressively. But even then, some horses were left with permanent neurological damage. And worse... no, *infinitely* more worse...some horses still perished despite medical intervention.

Let's not go there yet, Cal silently acknowledged, his lips pulled in tight.

"Maya's on her way," Cathy said as she slowly jogged toward him. At ten feet out, she gasped and bent down to grab her knees, her face ghostly pale as she breathed laboriously.

"Are you okay?" Cal asked, his head swiveling back and forth between Molly and Cathy.

She nodded, still bent over. "Just not used to moving this quick anymore, I guess."

"Try and take it easy," he said, knowing well that the current situation made that next to impossible. He waited a moment for Cathy to slowly straighten up, then said, "I'm bringing Molly into the barn. She has her own stall—right?"

"Yes, but there's an empty double box stall that might make it easier to work around her."

"Good—let's bring her in there."

"Is she going to be okay?" Jeremy asked as he approached Cal while he and Cathy slowly walked Molly to the barn. Cal was about to tell him to back away, then stopped. "Just stay on this side of me," he said gently, gesturing to his left side, as his right side faced Molly. She was in too compromised of a state to dangerously act out at this point, but as Cal saw the fear and concern in Jeremy's eyes, he momentarily held his breath. The last thing he wanted to do was make a promise he couldn't keep.

"We're going to do everything we can to help her," he said, doubling down on reassurance in his voice. The statement was true—it was the outcome that was still up for grabs.

Cal had nearly completed a thorough physical exam of Molly when Cathy called out from her surveillance spot at the barn entrance. "Maya's here!"

Cal felt a surge of relief flow through him. It wasn't just from knowing there would now be two veterinary experts weighing in on Molly's condition. It was a recognition that Maya's presence *did* something to him. He wasn't sure exactly what, but only knew that he felt an unusual sense of *everything is going to be okay* when she was near.

"I got here as soon as I could," she said as she entered the stall, voice calm but eyes registering deep concern.

As Jeremy ran to her and threw his arms around her waist in a tight hug, Cal watched as she winced in pain from her still-tender ribs. "It's okay, honey," she said soothingly. "We're going to do everything we can for Molly."

Her eyes immediately locked on to Cal's. "Cathy gave me a rundown of Molly's symptoms on the drive over. What are you thinking? EPM?"

He nodded. "I assume she was vaccinated for triple E, West Nile and rabies—right?"

"Yes, in late May," Maya said quietly as she continued to closely examine Molly. She turned to Cathy. "How was she this morning?"

"Perfectly fine." Cathy's voice was laden with disbelief. "Whatever this is, it came on suddenly."

Maya took a deep breath, matching the tightness that Cal felt in his own chest. "That does make me question whether she had some kind of head injury."

Cal nodded, turning to Cathy. "You mentioned she was bullied by the other horses before you put her in a separate pasture. Is it possible she was kicked in the head or fell?"

Cathy shook her head. "I watched the whole interaction. It looked like Moxie got a nip in on Molly's rump when she turned to run off, but that's it. I immediately put her in her own turnout after that."

Maya glanced at Cal, her face strained. He knew there was a twofold reason for her angst. Concern for Molly, of course, but also for Jeremy, who was now bearing witness to a horse in neurological distress. He looked over as the young boy stood silently by, only the brief wringing of his hands indicating the true depth of his worry for the stricken mare. Should they ask him to wait outside? Cal pondered the thought for a quick moment, until recalling how he, too, had insisted on being present as a boy whenever the vet came around for a sick horse.

Cal let go of the breath that he'd been holding, reminding himself that as both a vet and a mother, Maya clearly knew what she was doing. If she felt Jeremy should be somewhere else right now, she'd have said as much.

Instead, he watched as she reached over and squeezed Jeremy's balled-up hand, looking into his eyes and holding on until his fingers relaxed. "You okay? You can wait in the truck while we—"

"No," Jeremy forcibly interjected, his eyes pleading with her. "I want to stay. *Please*."

Maya nodded, her tightened lips working overtime to push out a smile.

She turned to Cal, her eyes fraught with emotion, but her voice all business. "Let's draw some blood for serological testing, and do a spinal tap."

Cathy, who had been standing several feet away, her face grim with concern, broke her silence. "Can you detect EPM in the blood and spinal fluid?"

"Not the actual parasite, but antibodies from exposure," Cal explained. "If the exposure is very recent, there might not be any antibodies yet. If that's the case, we can retest in a week or two."

He gripped Molly's halter and steadied her with a firm hand on the outer right side of her neck as Maya rubbed an alcohol swab on the left side of the neck that faced them. She inserted the needle deftly into a vein, her turquoise cast in full view as she girded her left hand just above Molly's shoulder, then pulled back on the plunger. Crimson-red blood instantly pooled into the chamber.

The next fluid withdrawal would not be as easy. Spinal fluid could be collected from the cervical neck area or the back lumbar region of a horse, with the former method requiring general anesthesia and the latter standing sedation only. Opting for the less risky procedure—especially in the context of a stall versus a hospital setting—Maya administered an IV injection of detomidine hydrochloride, followed by a localized injection of lidocaine hydrochloride to numb the withdrawal area.

Once the sedative had taken hold, Cal shaved and cleaned a triangular patch between the L6 and S1 vertebrae, then palpated the juncture between the bones. As he slowly inserted an 18-gauge, six-inch-long needle into the spinal canal, Molly arched her back, a normal reaction to pressure that could still be felt despite adequate sedation.

The fluid withdrawal now complete, he handed the vial to Maya, her look of relief matching his own.

"Nicely done," she said, her eyes meeting his and conveying that the compliment was more than one vet admiring the skills of another. Perhaps she sensed his emotional involvement in Molly's plight, a shared desire to save the mare no matter what it took, but also a keen awareness of how Molly's fate would impact Jeremy. He'd worked with many other equine vets over the years, got along perfectly fine with most of them—a few know-it-alls being the exception—but never did he feel a deeper connection with a colleague like he felt now with Maya.

She carefully placed the vial in the carrying case next to the blood sample, then turned to Cathy, who'd been viewing the procedure from the far end of the stall. "I'll get this sent off to the lab ASAP."

"Do we wait for results before starting any medication?" Cathy asked.

"With suspected EPM, we typically start treating right away. Especially when the symptoms are this pronounced. The thing with testing is that it's not one hundred percent conclusive—even with the gold standard of testing both blood and spinal fluid, rather than just the blood."

Maya turned to Cal. "Do you agree?"

"Absolutely." Looking into Maya's soulful eyes, she could say that the moon was made of green cheese and he'd wholeheartedly agree. But take the mesmerizing effects of her presence out of the equation, and her treatment assessment was still entirely spot-on.

"This is ponazuril paste," Maya said, handing several tubes to Cathy. "Each tube contains seven days of treatment, but we'll start her on a triple loading dose today."

"How long will she be on this for?" Cathy asked.

"The normal course is twenty-eight days. It does cross the blood-brain barrier to directly target the parasite, but doesn't completely eradicate it. But what it doesn't get, Molly's immune system should be able to kick in and finish off."

"Hopefully," Cathy said quietly, reaching over to stroke Molly's flaxen mane. "The fact that she's even let me touch her right now is hard to believe."

Cal, too, had made a mental note of Molly's sudden transformation from skittish to subdued. Was it a side effect of her neurological impairment? He couldn't be sure. Or maybe she knew they were trying to help her. It wouldn't be the first time he'd witnessed an untrusting, hard-to-control horse turn docile when its life depended on human intervention.

"We'll also give her an injection of Banamine today, and I'll leave some Banamine paste with you to continue treating for seven days," Maya said, a syringe of the medication already in hand. A quick swab of Molly's neck, and it was administered within seconds.

"Do you have vitamin E on hand?" Cal asked.

Cathy nodded. "I do."

"You'll want to start her on a high dose of ten thousand IU per day."

Cathy raised her eyebrows. "Wow—that *is* high."

"I know," Cal conceded, "but it can help counteract some of the oxidative stress that EPM can cause."

"Well," Cathy began, lips curved upward into a wry smile. "Far be it for me to question advice from a Hunk for Horses."

Maya spit out a laugh at Cathy's tension-breaking comment. Cal chuckled as well, but his brief laughter ended as he spotted Jeremy out of the corner of his eye. Maya turned to Jeremy as well, as though sensing Cal's concern.

"You doing okay?" he asked as walked over to the far end of the stall and kneeled down next to him.

Jeremy nodded solemnly. "She's really sick, isn't she?"

Cal knew he needed to strike a balance between truthfulness and hope. But as he looked into Jeremy's distressed eyes, he felt compelled to let the pendulum swing more toward hope. "Yes, but your mom and I are doing everything to help her get better. And Cathy, too."

Out in the parking area, Cal approached Maya as she was straightening out supplies in the back of her work truck. "Need help with anything?"

She turned to him and smiled. "I'm good, thanks."

The sun caught golden highlights in her hair that he hadn't noticed before. He stared at her, both realizing he shouldn't be so obvious—and also not caring. Well, he *did* care...but not enough to look away. With her delicate features and petite, lithe body, she could easily be mistaken for a ballerina. Albeit...a ballerina in jeans, mud boots and a ponytail with a couple of wood shavings tacked on to the ends.

Cal held in a snicker at the thought, though he couldn't completely put the brakes on a smile.

Maya viewed him from slightly narrowed eyes. "What's so funny?"

"Nothing," he lied, knowing she would probably welcome the comparison to a ballerina like he would to a...well, the same. *I never did look good in tights...*

But Maya, however, in a dainty tutu? She'd knock that look out of the park. Even so, he'd take her natural, outdoorsy appearance over something so frilly and contrived any day of the week—hair shavings and all.

"Are we going home now?" Jeremy asked as he walked over, cutting into Cal's very enjoyable thoughts.

"I'm going to drop the sample vials off at FedEx on the way, and then we'll head back home," Maya replied as she shut the truck doors and turned to him. "And how about we make it a pizza night? I'll put an order in for delivery, extra cheese and mushrooms—your favorite. How's that sound?"

Jeremy looked up at her, his eyes widened. "Can Cal come over, too?"

Maya visibly stiffened at the question, but Cal couldn't blame her. He was feeling bunged up by the unexpected inquiry as well. Her eyes darted over to him, and they certainly weren't saying, *I'd love for you to join us.* More like, *I'd love if you could get me out of this predicament right now.* And so he did.

"I actually have plans tonight. But thanks." He forced a smile. "And enjoy the dinner. You can never go wrong when pizza's on the menu."

Seeing the near relief in Maya's eyes was hard to take, but Cal reminded himself there was a reason for her reaction. Her immediate nuclear family consisted of herself and Jeremy, and it was a tight-knit, treasured cocoon that had no room for an outsider like him.

Is that what I am? An outsider?

Cal's breath caught in his throat. Why was he even asking himself this? It wasn't a question he'd ever posed to himself before. And if he had, the answer would have been, *Yes, I am, thank you very much.* No shame. No regrets. No thought that it ever could be…or should be…anything different. The harsh reality clashed with what he felt had been a growing closeness as they worked in tandem earlier on Molly. Did he just imagine a deeper connection?

"Cal?"

Cal snapped back to attention as Maya's voice penetrated his runaway train of thought. "Sorry—did you say something?"

"Just that I'm on emergency call tonight, so I'll be looking in on Molly if things take a turn for the worse. But the fact that we got her started on ponazuril as soon as her symptoms were spotted… I feel reasonably confident that we caught things just in time."

Cal smiled and nodded. If he had displayed his true feelings, the smile would be curved downward…or flatlined, at the very least. Not that he didn't want to share Maya's optimism. But he'd seen enough of "things are looking good" scenarios that had boomeranged over the course of a night, to know that when it came to equine medicine, things could change on a dime. Still, he'd do his best to stay positive.

"Well, I guess I'll be heading out." It was hard to conjure up a smile after everything that had happened earlier at Happy Hooves, but for Jeremy's sake, he managed to flash one his way. "Thanks for helping out today. You did good. Especially alerting us to the fact that something was off with Molly."

Maya peered down proudly at her son, then back to Cal. As she locked eyes with him, he wondered what she was thinking. It had to be *something*, because instead of looking away, she held his gaze. In fact…if he didn't know any better, it almost seemed as though she was having second thoughts about including him for dinner. *Almost*.

Then again, he reasoned, it had been a long, stressful day, and his powers of perception were probably not fully up to par.

Climbing into his truck, he waved out the window at Maya and Jeremy, then headed down the long, pebble-strewn driveway.

* * *

Maya watched as Cal's truck rambled past her and continued down the driveway. Moments later, it turned right onto the main road, then disappeared from view. She continued to stare straight ahead, trying to steady her roller-coaster thoughts. If she could will his truck backward like a reverse tractor beam, would she do so? That she was even posing this question to herself was just one step short of shocking.

You don't do casual. You know this. Don't cross professional boundaries, and you and Jeremy will avoid getting attached.

She turned to look at Jeremy, his solemn face grabbing her hard in the gut. She couldn't assume it had anything to do with Cal driving off...could she?

Perhaps he was lamenting Molly's situation. They were all feeling it. A beautiful mare, on the cusp of coming out of her shell, who was now facing a potentially deadly condition.

"Come on," she said to Jeremy as she squeezed his shoulder. "Jenna's coming by to feed everyone tonight, but how about we stop by the clinic and check in on the gang before heading home."

Jeremy looked up at her and nodded, the hint of a smile on his face. It wasn't much, but she'd take it. Because there was one other reason she could be smiling right now...and she just sent him away to eat a lonely dinner by himself.

CHAPTER FIVE

MAYA GRIPPED THE steering wheel of her truck as it hit a shallow pothole on a poorly lit back road in the town of Porterville. Twenty minutes earlier, she'd been roused from a relatively sound sleep after receiving a page from the Equine Associates after-hours answering service. It wasn't about Molly, who was now three days into her treatment, but rather a horse who had become cast in its stall. The most typical way that a horse became cast was when it rolled on the ground and up against a stall wall, rendering it unable to get back up on its feet.

As prey animals, horses panicked when they found themselves in such a vulnerable state, and Maya had seen more than her share of the self-inflicted injuries—sometimes grave—that resulted from a horse trying to kick its way free.

Which was why she was now wide awake and relieved that her GPS indicated she was one minute out from her destination. Turning onto a narrow dirt driveway, Maya drove up to a small parking area, her focused and alert eyes popping open to maximum width.

It can't be... she thought as she spotted what looked like Cal's truck directly in front of her headlights. Realizing how common dark blue trucks were in the area, Maya shook her head at the silliness of jumping to such an improbable conclusion.

Cal on the mind much?

Swinging the door open to her own truck, she quickly hopped out and gasped as she face-planted into something very solid.

"Whoa!" a familiar voice said as two strong hands reached out to steady her by the shoulders.

Her face now removed from Cal's chest, Maya looked up, eyes wider than the nearly full moon that hovered overhead. "Cal! What are you doing here?"

He greeted her with a smile and a minimal reply. "Helping you."

Maya shook her head in confusion. Something—no, *lots* of things—were not adding up. "How'd you know there's an emergency? The answering service has our schedule—that's why they called me tonight, not you."

"I asked them to notify me as well on your nights."

Maya's confusion was growing. "Wait…what?"

"Maya, your arm's still in a cast, and I'm going to hedge my bets that your ribs aren't fully healed yet, either. If you're going to pull up a kicking, one-thousand-pound horse, you're going to need my help."

He looked down at her cast-covered arm, and it was only then that Maya realized he was still holding on to her. There was no danger of her falling at this point, so she knew she should pull away. Except…*let's just stay here a little bit longer.*

As Cal locked eyes with her, he seemed equally unwilling to let go. "I mean, how in the world were you planning to do this on your own?" he asked softly.

She knew he had a point, but couldn't fully shelve her stubbornness. "If I couldn't do it with the owners' help, I was going to call the volunteer fire department."

He stared hard at her for several moments, and she couldn't tell if he was annoyed by her answer, or impressed. Maybe it was a little of both. Slowly, he broke into a smile. "I'm the only volunteer you'll need tonight."

Reminding herself that time was of the essence in any emergency, she took a step back and gently slipped out of his embrace. "I'm not sure what to say. Other than thank-you."

He grinned. "No need to thank me. Now, let's go save a horse."

Twenty minutes later, the grateful owners of Buttercup, a palomino mare, effusively thanked Maya and Cal as they all headed out of the barn. Cal wrapped up the rope that he and Maya had tied to Buttercup's lower legs in order to flip her over and away from the stall wall, enabling her to rise up on her own.

Walking to their vehicles, Maya thanked Cal again. He'd been right—how *would* she have been able to pull Buttercup up on her own? It was a reminder that even though she truly believed the human brain was the strongest muscle when interacting with horses, it certainly didn't hurt to have some brute strength on hand in physically challenging situations like this.

Arriving at their trucks, Maya paused as her pager vibrated against her hip. She pulled it off her belt and read the text.

"A colic case in Dearbon." She looked up at Cal, who had halted beside her. "This is so weird how emergencies seem to happen all at once. We'll go weeks without a single call, and then there'll be several in one night."

Cal looked up at the night sky. "No full moon, but I know what you mean. I've seen the same thing happen at other practices."

Standing oh-so-close to Cal, Maya could do little more in this moment than stare into his eyes. Because, well...why not? There might not be a full moon, but there was enough of a crescent glow to capture their unique hue. His gaze latched on to hers, and she felt something shoot through the entirety of her body. Electricity? Moonbeams? A combination of both?

With an eye squeeze and a headshake, she forcibly extracted herself from the almost hypnotic pull that Cal...or his eyes, or the moment itself...had on her.

An emergency was unfolding, and she needed to leave *now*.

Maya pulled her truck keys out of her jacket

pocket. "Well, thanks again for your help. I'll see you in the morning."

Cal seemed almost amused by her announcement. He raised his eyebrows, lips twisted to one side as he flashed her a look that said, *Really?*

"Sorry—you can't get rid of me that easy."

Maya's heart skipped a beat, until it fully registered that he was strictly talking about emergency visits.

She shook her head. "No—I'm on call tonight, not you. Go home and get some rest."

"I'm already here, and there's no way I'm going back to bed when there's a horse who needs my help." With a twinkle in his eye, he nodded to Maya's cast-covered arm. "And perhaps a veterinarian who does, too."

Maya opened her mouth to protest, but nothing came out. Which both frustrated and surprised her. How could she say no to Cal's help, when they made such a good team?

It was nearly 4:00 a.m. when Maya and Cal walked back to their trucks in the Shady Acres Farm parking lot.

Zeus, an off-the-track Thoroughbred, was resting comfortably in his stall after an acute colic episode that had required pumping mineral oil into his stomach through a tube that had been inserted into his nose and snaked down into his gut.

"Another happy ending," Maya said, her voice sounding as fatigued as the rest of her. She opened the back of her truck and began loading equipment back into its place.

"My favorite kind," Cal said as he stood next to her. "Here, let me." He picked up a large metal pail with tubing and a hefty jug of mineral oil, and placed them back in their spots under a shelf on the right.

"I can lift that, you know," Maya said, not sure whether to be more annoyed or appreciative of his gallant gesture.

Cal casually shrugged, his reply equally nonchalant. "I know you can."

A simple observation, and yet one that prompted Maya to recall all the times that Max had taken the opposite stance, standing back and watching her struggle to lift something heavy. "You don't need special treatment," he'd say. Which had been true. *And yet...*

The recollections quickly shifted the scales in favor of appreciation for Cal's kindness.

Five minutes later, everything was packed up, and Maya closed the back of the truck. She turned to Cal, slightly unnerved to find that he'd been staring at her.

Say something, she chided herself—anything to override the awkwardness she felt.

She opted for a truthful observation. "At this point, I'm tired, but still wide-awake, if you know what I mean."

"I do." Cal cocked his head to the side, continuing to watch Maya intently. "You know, we're not far from my cabin. How about if I make us some breakfast? I don't have any maple syrup, but I've got coffee and..."

Oh boy, oh boy, oh boy, oh boy...

Maya's gulp nearly caught in her parched throat.

"Breakfast bars?" he continued in a questioning tone.

Another hard swallow. "What about them?"

"I have some," Cal said, a one-sided grin forming. "Blueberry strudel, I think. And coffee. Which I already said, but I'm repeating because I know it's your thing."

It was. But still, she couldn't answer.

Even under his jacket, Maya could see Cal's chest—his *fantastic* chest, which she imagined must be rippling with muscles—heave with...something. Anticipation? Exasperation?

Just keep heaving, she thought, before forcing herself to pry her eyes away.

Cal let out a slight sigh. "Look, I know what you said about colleagues not crossing the line. But this isn't a date. It's more like two tired vets who worked together all night to save some horses, just kicking back with a cup of coffee to reenergize and get ready for another day's work." He glanced at his watch. "It might still be dark now, but not for long."

Nope, thought Maya. *I can't do this. And I'm just going to tell it to him straight.*

She held her breath for a moment, then gave her answer. "Okay."

Cal grinned, his eyes wide with surprise.

I know how you feel, Maya wanted to say, wondering how the *no* in her brain had turned into a *yes* when it had exited her mouth.

"Follow me," Cal said as he nodded toward his truck.

As Maya watched Cal walk to his truck with an unassuming swagger...replaying all the ways he'd helped her tonight despite no obligation to do so... she wondered no more why *no* had been flipped on its head.

Colleagues just kicking back with coffee to reenergize for another day's work. I can't believe she bought that line.

Cal stopped short of letting out a *whoop whoop!* as he waited for Maya to pull her truck up behind his. She flashed her headlights, and he pulled out onto the main road.

Fifteen minutes later, he held the front door open to his cabin and waited for Maya to enter. As she passed by him, just inches away, he half closed his eyes as an enticing scent traveled with her like a portable floral breeze. How could anyone smell literally as fresh as a daisy after a full night of physically grueling work?

You can ponder that later. Because right now, his only concern was not screwing up the opportunity to get to know Maya better.

"Wow, this place is great," she said as she admired the cabin's rustic charm.

"Isn't it?" Cal agreed. "I guess for the rich guy who owns it, this is the equivalent of a tiny house that he visits once or twice a year. But for me, there's lots of space and a great loft upstairs. Plus, the deck." He nodded to the front of the cabin before rummaging through the cabinets for coffee and breakfast bars.

"I have a deck on my house, too. Well, more like a wraparound porch. But I can't imagine not having a spot like that to sit outside and just take in the peacefulness of nature."

Cal turned on the coffee maker and waited several seconds for the first percolating gurgle before turning back to Maya. "Glad you feel that way, because I thought we could have coffee out on the deck and watch the sun come up."

She stared at him, her expression momentarily frozen.

"Or...not," Cal said slowly.

Maya gave a quick shake of the head, as though tossing off her cautious hesitation. "No, that's fine."

Seated on the deck a short time later, Maya looked out to the purplish-black sky that hovered over the distant mountaintops.

"I'm sure you've seen your share of beautiful sunrises, given that you've lived all over the world," she said reflectively.

"I have. But the sunsets here have been pretty

awesome. And sharing them with someone makes them that much more amazing."

Maya swung her head in his direction, a look on her face that said, *Did you just say that?*

He did, and it was a surprise to him, too. Not that he didn't actually feel this way, especially when—no, make that *only* when—this *someone* was Maya. But he had to be careful about oversharing his attraction to her. At least for the time being, given that he couldn't be sure where he fell in her eyes on the romantic spectrum of *not a chance in hell* on one end, and *I'm open to the possibility* on the other.

"Does Jeremy know when you leave during the night for an emergency?" A genuine question, but also the chance to redirect the conversation.

"It depends. I don't like to wake him on a school night, since he needs his sleep. But I might if I think there's a chance I'll still be gone when he gets up. I do text Carla, though. She lives in an apartment above my garage, and looks after Jeremy when I'm at work." Maya paused to take a sip of coffee, looking out wistfully as streaks of lighter violet emerged seemingly out of nowhere in the sky. "Pretty soon, he won't need anyone watching over him so closely. It's hard to believe how quickly he's growing up."

Cal smiled. He could almost viscerally feel Maya's love for her son. It was the way that it should be, even if his own experience was devoid of any such maternal bond.

"He's a great kid, and a natural around horses."

Maya seemed pleased by the observation. "Between my genes and his father's, I don't think he has a choice." She paused, as though wondering whether to say more. "You probably know from the picture in the office that he was a horse vet, too. He died when Jeremy was three years old."

Cal thought back to how he had assumed that Maya and her former husband were divorced. The tragic reality was so much more devastating, and he winced at the thought of what she must have gone through. "I'm so sorry, Maya."

She acknowledged his sympathy with a pained but appreciative smile. "I always tell myself that he died doing what he loved. He was heading out during the night to an emergency call and was hit by a drunk driver." Maya paused for several moments. "It was my night for emergencies, and he insisted on going instead."

"I'm sure he'd make that same decision all over again," he said quietly. He didn't know the man, but he *did* know—or was at least getting to know—Maya, and there was no way she wasn't harboring some undeserved guilt about how things had played out on that fateful night.

"You're probably right." Maya bent forward to pick up a breakfast bar off the plate, then took a bite. "Not bad," she said, an obvious attempt to segue into a less emotionally charged conversation topic.

Cal figured she'd have said the same if it tasted like cardboard—anything to change the subject. He readily played along, scooping up a breakfast bar and taking a good-sized bite. "Better than if I baked them myself, I can tell you that."

Maya laughed, and Cal felt his shoulders loosen up with relief. It was good to see her finally relax.

"Look," he said, pointing to the first golden rays that were peeking through the treetops to the east. "The sun's just starting to rise."

"Beautiful," Maya said softly. "The start of another day."

Cal lifted his mug of coffee and raised it in a toast. "To an even-keel, emergency-free day."

Maya grinned as she lightly clanged her mug against his. "I'll sip to that."

Their eyes met, and his gaze dropped to her lips. If he leaned in now and kissed those sweet, lovely lips…would she meet him halfway? A *quarter* of the way? Would she throw up a hand and stop him in his tracks?

Time stood still as more potential scenarios raced through his mind. She'd kiss him back hard. No—it would be a soft kiss…soft and lingering.

Wait. She had made it clear that she didn't want to cross that line, so maybe she'd kick him in the…

Bzzzzzzzzzzzz

Maya's vibrating pager pierced the silence, prompting both of them to jerk up straight in their chairs. For a split second, Cal wanted to thank the pager for putting the brakes on his dizzying over-analysis of a kiss. *What ever happened to simply seizing the moment?* But then, reality set in. If the pager was buzzing, then an emergency was heating up somewhere.

Maya pulled the pager from her belt clip, pausing to meet Cal's eyes. It was a momentary hesitation, but enough to convey to him that she knew where his thoughts had been heading. As in right smack onto her lips. Had her thoughts been going in the same direction? Cal couldn't tell, but right now, they needed to focus on other things.

"It's Molly," Maya said, looking up from the pager message, gray eyes clouded with concern.

Cal lurched from the chair. "Let's go."

He held out his hand to help Maya to her feet, but she was already standing. A moment of hesitation, then she reached out and clasped his hand. The touch lasted for only a second…actually three—yes, he was counting—but he'd take it in lieu of a kiss. To him, it was a sign of growing trust, and right now, that trumped everything.

CHAPTER SIX

"I'M SORRY. I know it's early," Cathy said as Maya and Cal exited the truck in the Happy Hooves parking area. Her eyes were both anxious and fatigued, and Maya wondered if she'd been making around-the-clock checks on Molly.

"That's okay," Maya said. "It's been a busy night for emergencies, so we were already up."

"What's going on?" Cal asked, a calmness in his voice that Maya knew masked his concern.

"She's having what looks like a seizure."

Maya didn't like the sound of that, and judging from the look on Cal's face, neither did he. "I'll get some phenobarbital," he said, heading to the truck.

"When did it start?" Maya asked.

"I'm not sure. Tonight was the first night that I didn't sleep out in the barn since this started. I mean, she seemed to be responding to the medication, so I thought we were out of the danger zone."

Hearing the distress in Cathy's voice, Maya reached over and gently squeezed her arm. "It's okay. You were right to think that."

Cathy drew in a deep breath as she allowed Maya's reassurance to sink in.

"But when I woke up at five thirty," she continued, "the first thing I did was head out to check on her. She was down in the stall, her whole body was just like…quivering. I called right away."

"I'm glad you did."

"In all my years, I've never seen a horse have a seizure before and it's…" Cathy's voice cracked before it dropped off altogether.

"I know," Maya said softly. "It's hard to witness, but just know that Molly is most likely completely unaware of what her body is doing, and isn't in any pain."

"It doesn't look that way," Cathy said, her voice slightly choked. "But I know they say the same when people have seizures. Do you know why this is happening?"

"EPM targets the spinal cord and brain, and that can lead to seizures."

"Even after the start of medication?"

This question wasn't so easy to answer. Maya had treated her share of EPM cases over the years, and when caught early like it had been with Molly, the disease typically didn't progress to seizures. But there were so many mitigating factors that played into the disease—into *any* disease—that Maya knew she could only make an educated guess at best.

"Ready?" Cal asked as he headed toward them, an injectable syringe in one hand and a carrying case with emergency supplies in the other.

Maya hadn't yet answered Cathy's question, but it would have to wait. The trio quickly headed to the barn, with Cal entering first into the stall. Molly was lying flat on her side, eyes closed and her entire body twitching wildly. He knelt down beside her, with Maya quickly dropping to her knees next to him.

Cathy was right, Maya thought. It was hard to see a horse in the throes of a seizure, even as an experienced vet. She briefly held her breath as Cal placed a hand on the mare's shoulder, sweeping upward to palpate the jugular vein in her neck. Maya watched closely as he injected the needle, pulling back on the plunger for the telltale sign of blood that he was in the vein, then administering the medication.

Almost instantly, the full-body twitching began to subside. Only when it stopped altogether did Maya feel it was safe to breathe.

Cal turned to her, relief in his eyes as he locked on to her gaze. But Molly wasn't out of the woods yet. In higher doses, phenobarbital was an effective sedative strong enough to function as anesthesia, but that wasn't its purpose today. They needed for Molly to fully come around and get back on her feet. Only then would Maya feel that Molly still had a fighting chance, and judging from Cal's furrowed brow, she knew he felt the same.

A minute passed, and then another. As Molly finally blinked open her eyes, Maya grabbed Cal's forearm in a mix of relief and excitement, then quickly let go.

Hands off the hunky vet, she reminded herself.

But the look in Cal's eyes as she released her grip—the same longing gaze that she had seen during their almost-kiss at his cabin—made it clear that the directive was hers alone. In fact, she half expected him to say *Hands* on *the vet, please?*

As Molly began to stir, Maya decided to shelve that thought for another time.

"That's it, girl," Cal said soothingly as Molly lifted her head.

It pained Maya to see how her head was still tilted to the right, a stark reminder of how EPM could wreak havoc on a horse's body through a myriad of neurological impairments. Hopefully, this symptom—along with the others—would improve as the treatment took hold. But Maya wasn't kidding herself. She knew Molly had a long road ahead of her. And right now, it wasn't clear if this was a journey she could even make. All it would take was another seizure and…

Maya bit down on her bottom lip to derail her worrisome thoughts. She looked up at Cal and immediately felt better. Where there was angst in her eyes, there was reassurance in his. *We'll help Molly get through this together.* And for the first time in years, she felt it wasn't such a bad thing having another vet by her side to help tackle a tough case.

"Oh, thank god!" Cathy exclaimed from just outside the stall as Molly kicked her forelegs out in front of her, then heaved herself up into a full stand.

"I second that!" Maya replied, exchanging a relieved glance with Cal.

He blew out a puff of air, then shook his head with a smile that widened from ear to ear. "I don't know about you, but I think I just held my breath for two minutes straight."

"Same here," Maya said, relief in her voice.

"I'm going to get some more shavings, make things nice and comfy for her," Cathy said.

Alone with Cal, Maya fought the urge to hug him over their shared relief that Molly was still hanging on. As she looked up at him, he reached over and brushed a lock of hair away from her eyes. "That was a close one," he said quietly, surprise registering on his face as Maya briefly clasped his hand before letting go.

Still, with Cal just inches away, she closed her eyes, leaning into the moment...both wishing that it was...and glad that it wasn't...more. A conflicting wish, true, but she had her guarded heart to thank for that.

A loud snort from Molly snapped Maya out of her dreamy state, her shared moment with Cal paused as together they turned to the mare and grappled with the latest setback. The lab test results that she'd received the night before confirmed EPM. But if that was true, why wasn't Molly responding quicker to the treatment?

"I wonder if the issue is that coming from out

West, she hasn't had the same exposure to the parasite," Cal said, as if reading her thoughts.

"Yes," Maya replied, quickly realizing that he was onto something. "In fact, not long ago I read up on a study that showed most horses in New England have been exposed to Sarcocystis neurona. Most never develop EPM symptoms, but they have a heightened immunity to the disease if they're ever exposed to it again. Molly most likely had zero immunity built up, so she's been hit that much harder."

"We may just need to give things more time," Cal said. "Let's stay the course, and hopefully things will start to turn around."

Outside the barn entrance, Cathy approached with a bag of shavings, which she promptly dropped to the ground before lobbing a teasing question at Cal.

"So are you ready for the Hunks for Horses fundraiser next weekend?" she asked, followed by a wink in Maya's direction.

"Is it that soon?" Cal replied beleagueredly, though he grinned just the same.

Maya let out a faint chuckle, which she quickly squelched as the image of Susie and her long, fluttering eyelashes flashed in her mind. No doubt she'd be just one of many overeager bidders at the event, all hankering to win a date with Cal. Which meant *someone* would soon be cozying up to dinner with him…but it wouldn't be Maya. She'd made sure of that right off the bat, buying a half dozen tickets from Cathy the day after Cal had been roped into participating—and insisting her name not be entered into the drawing.

"Afraid you might get paired with Santa Claus or the meerkat?" Cathy had asked at the time.

"No," Maya had said with a wry smirk. "Just want to steer clear of any complications in my life."

Cathy had raised a knowing eyebrow at the time, and as far as Maya was concerned, no further explanation was needed. Still...it didn't hurt to remind both present parties of her "leave me out of this" intentions.

"You put my tickets aside so they won't be added to the draw—right?"

"Of course," Cathy said, eyes wide and a smile so stilted that it looked like it had been propped open with invisible toothpicks as stilts.

"You're not going to be entered into the draw?" Cal asked, his elbow shooting out into Cathy's side. She hopped with a yelp, then resumed her wooden smile.

Maya narrowed her eyes at him. "Why are you nudging Cathy?"

Cal lifted his bent arm and stared at his elbow. "I did? Huh. It must've been a knee-jerk reaction."

"You mean an elbow-jerk," Cathy nervously corrected him.

Cal greeted her observation with a plastered smile. "Right."

Eyes further tapered to near slits, Maya looked at Cathy, then back to Cal. "You two are acting weird."

"Me?" they asked in unison.

"Yes, you. *Both* of you." Her sigh turned into a smile. "Well, call us if you need anything, Cathy."

"I will."

Maya looked at Cal, waiting for him to join her on the walk back to their ride. "You coming?"

"Actually, I'll meet you at the truck."

Maya's hackles were now raised to the point that they nearly lifted her off the ground. "Okayyyyy…"

"I need to talk to Cathy about what I should wear for the fundraiser," Cal further explained. Or so he apparently thought.

Maya twisted her mouth to the side, a *Yeah, right!* expression doing the talking for her.

"Seriously!" Cal exclaimed. "And I want it to be a surprise for you, too. Even though you're not actively participating in the name draw." He turned to Cathy. "I'm thinking maybe there might be some kind of sexy male vet costume like those female nurse ones, but I have other ideas, too."

"Fine," Maya said, shrugging her shoulders. "Just make sure it's something Susie will like."

She capped her observation off with a teasing-slash-bratty smile, and headed for the truck.

"That can't be the same Susie…"

Cal didn't let Cathy finish the question. "I have to make this quick," he said, one eye on Maya's truck across the way. "You never did answer me about calling Maya's name out in the drawing."

"How could I? Jeremy came running into the barn about Molly."

"I know." Cal softened his voice. He normally wasn't this relentless about...*anything*...but there was so much riding on Cathy's answer.

"What I didn't have a chance to tell you is what Maya just mentioned herself. She doesn't want to be entered in the draw."

Cal sighed, his shoulders slumping under the weight of defeat.

Cathy looked up, twisting her jaw as she silently pondered. "Although..."

Boom. Cal stood up straight, renewed with hope before he even knew what Cathy was about to propose.

"Oh, this is good," she said, shaking her head with a devious chuckle.

"Tell me!"

"Remember how I told you my niece takes care of social media for the rescue?"

Cal nodded, wondering where she could possibly be going with this.

"Well—and how do I say this nicely about my sister's daughter—she's a screwup."

Cal nearly choked on his amusement. "*What?*"

"Oh, you know how the younger generation is these days. Eyes glued twenty-four seven to their phones, unable to follow directions that a pet rat could master in two seconds. I know Maya's heard me gripe about how many times Charlene's messed things up, or forgot to post something that she promised to take care of. I put up with it because I can only afford to pay her peanuts, and so far, she's not made an issue of it."

Cal grinned. "That's what family's for."

Cathy half rolled her eyes. "I suppose."

"This is pretty funny...but I'm still not sure what this has to do with explaining to Maya how her name ended up being called at the drawing."

Cathy grinned. "I'm getting to that. All I have to do is tell her that Charlene was in charge of tickets, and that I told her to put Maya's aside and *not* add them to the bucket. In fact, I probably won't have to say any more than that, because she'll instantly assume Charlene messed that task up, too."

A smile slowly worked its way from ear to ear. "Cathy, you are brilliant."

"Stop flirting with me," Cathy pretend-growled, though her eyes added a one-word caveat: *Not*.

CHAPTER SEVEN

CAL STARED INTO the full-length bathroom mirror, then shook his head. That a rustic cabin would even have such a vanity contraption was one thing. But to be actually *using* it was another. And yet, here he was...turning his head from side to side to evaluate the angle of an Australian cowboy hat that rested on his head, and rolling his shirt sleeves up, then down, then up again.

Dude!

He stepped away from the mirror, irritated with himself, yet also on the verge of a chuckle. Had it really come to this? Preening in front of a mirror like a puffed-up peacock in the Aussie version of a Stetson, hoping to impress the girl? And not just *any* girl, mind you, but the one who'd been consuming his thoughts day and night. He hadn't *intended* for this to be the case, but the more time he spent around Maya, witnessing firsthand her fierce devotion to both her son and the horses in her care, it was impossible not to see that she was as beautiful on the inside as she was on the outside.

And now, he was a mere hour away from strutting across the stage at the Maplewood Grange, doing his best to feign surprise as Cathy called out Maya's name. And then what? Would Maya be glad for the "mistake" of having her name entered in the draw and landing a date with him? Furious instead? Cal sighed, realizing there was no point in overanalyzing the potential outcome. He'd find out soon enough.

Turning to leave the bathroom, he stopped and pivoted around to face the mirror once more. Tipping his hat, he murmured, "You got this, cowboy."

Then he rolled his eyes at himself and headed out the door.

Thirty minutes later, Cal peeked out from behind the thick stage curtains where he and the other fundraiser "horse hunks" had been milling about while waiting for the start of the draw. It was a full house, for sure, but there was only one audience member whose presence mattered to him.

Turning briefly back, Cal winced as the town sheriff lifted his plaid shirt out of his pants and patted a hairy stomach before rearranging the shirttails and tucking everything back in.

I didn't need to see that, he thought, before turning back to the mission at hand. Maya. He had to find where she was sitting. Not only to confirm she was here—even though she had promised when they had parted ways at the barn last night that she wouldn't miss the chance to witness his "Hunk for Horses debut," but also because just seeing her would put his mind at ease. And his body at…well, that was a thought that could wait for their date.

Suddenly, a hand shot up in the air. It was attached

to a forearm stacked high in bejeweled bracelets that nearly blinded him as they reflected the harsh fluorescent lights above.

"Cal!" exclaimed an unfortunately all-too-familiar voice. "I see you!"

Cal lurched his head back and pulled the curtain panels shut with white-knuckle ferocity. How in the world had Susie recognized his one eyeball sticking out of the tiny opening?

A tap on the back of his shoulder nearly sent him flying out of his cowboy boots.

"Whoa! Jumpy much?" Cathy asked, one eyebrow raised in amusement as he whirled around to face her.

He held his breath, then allowed a smirk to form. "Not usually, but I am tonight."

"I can see that." She leaned in with a conspiratorial whisper. "Relax. Everything's going according to plan."

"But I don't see Maya out there."

"Don't worry—she's here. She offered to help set up refreshments, so she might be in the kitchen. I'll make sure she takes a seat in time for the big surprise."

Glancing at her watch, Cathy looked up and clapped her hands twice. "Okay, guys. It's showtime! Remember, this is all to benefit the horses. So if you need to flex a muscle or two for the women…" Cathy paused, surveying the less-than-strapping participants who circled around her. "Or, um, flex your wonderful personalities, then go for it."

"*You* can show some muscle," she quipped out of the side of her mouth to Cal. He grinned, though there was only one woman he wanted to impress. And something told him Maya preferred the not-so-showboaty type.

I hope Cal shows some muscle, Maya thought as she took her seat toward the back of the room. Reminding herself that *someone* was going to end up on a date with him, and it wasn't going to be her, Maya did an about-face. *Okay, keep everything buttoned and zipped, please.* After all, there was no need to tempt herself with what she couldn't have.

Feeling slightly embittered over her earlier decision to sit out the actual draw, Maya reminded herself why it had to be this way.

He's leaving in less than two months. You already like him way more than is good for you. You think you can have a fling and not get attached, but girl... you know that's not true.

"Blah, blah, blah, blah, blah."

"I'm sorry—did you say something?" asked a woman seated next to Maya.

Maya's cheeks grew hot at the realization that she'd been talking gibberish out loud. "Oh—hi, Mrs. King. I was, uh, reciting my grocery list to myself." She forced a smile. "Helps me remember things."

"I do the same," Mrs. King said with a chuckle.

Dressed in a sharp navy-blue skirt suit, low-heeled shoes and with graying hair that was freshly curled and teased out into a lacquered helmet, the town seamstress—and fellow Maplewood Community Events Committee member—was at her usual regal best.

"Glad to see you here," Maya said, though substituting *surprised* for *glad* would probably be more accurate. "I can tell you firsthand that Happy Hooves Horse Rescue does some very important work."

"Well, I'm not much of a horse person, but I do try to support local charities."

Maya smiled. "Me too."

Mrs. King leaned in, her voice dropping down an octave. "Although, I have to say, when I got the flyer in the mail last week—that really sealed the deal for me."

Maya raised an eyebrow. "Oh?"

"Did you get a look at that horse vet who's in the draw?"

Maya's eyes bulged as the older woman licked her top lip and whispered, "Yummy."

The prim and proper Mrs. King...reduced to an overzealous admirer salivating on behalf of a Hunk for Horses. Maya let that sink in, concluding that she'd now officially seen it all.

"The flyer didn't mention what horse vet practice he works at. It's not yours—is it?"

Her jaw still partially ajar, Maya was relieved as Cathy took the stage to resounding applause that would've drowned out any potential answer. Maya pointed to the stage and clapped, nearly getting whacked in the head by a sturdy pocketbook as Mrs. King lifted her arms to join in the revelry.

One by one, Cathy introduced the Hunks...*er... participants*...drawing one name out of the bucket each time before moving on to the next.

When Susie's name was called, pairing her with Ed the Meerkat, Maya choked on a snicker. At least she was out of the running for Cal's draw, Maya thought, though poor Ed had no idea what he was in for. Judging from his ear-to-ear smile, however, he was more than game for whatever those monstrous eyelashes were bringing his way.

"And last but certainly not least," Cathy said into the handheld microphone after working her way through six back-to-back draws, "please give a hand for Cal Parker, our final Hunk for Horses participant tonight. Cal, do you have anything to say to this very eager audience?"

Cal lowered his head toward the microphone, dipping his hat as Maya swallowed hard. If ever there was a melding of gentlemanly manners with vibes that were sexy as...yeah, *that* word that rhymed with *muck*...then this was it.

"Just that I'm looking forward to my date with whoever is about to be picked from the bucket. And it means a lot to me knowing that the horses at Happy Hooves are benefiting from this very special event." He turned to Cathy. "Thanks for all you do."

Cathy's look of surprise was quickly followed up with a smile, and as she gestured with her free hand to Cal for the rapt audience, it took a moment for Maya to realize that her jaw was once again hovering just above the ground. But how else could she react when all around her, the normally staid townswomen—this was quaint, turn-back-the-clock Maplewood, after all—were practically climbing over each other to get to the ultimate prize?

Half expecting panties to start flying onto the stage, Maya could only hope that Mrs. King wasn't about to hike up her skirt and yank down a girdle.

Please...

But Maya's silent plea wasn't just about sparing herself a sight that would be hard to unsee. It was also an appeal to the universe.

Please don't let Cal like his chosen date too *much.*

Yes, it was a small and petty plea, Maya silently acknowledged, but she felt compelled to think it just the same.

"And the winner of a date with Cal is..."

Maya squeezed her eyes shut and dug her nails into her palm—anything to soften the blow.

"...Maya Evans!"

Maya opened her eyes, wondering why everyone was staring at her. For a second, she thought Cathy had called her name, but of course, that wasn't possible. Was there another Maya in the room? Maybe? Possibly?

"You lucky dog," Mrs. King whispered loudly in her ear as she leaned over.

Only then was Maya hit with reality. As Cal stared at her from the stage, a sexy, one-sided grin on his face, she revised that thought. A *smoldering, smoking-hot* reality. And a kind and compassionate one—qualities that might not be game changers for some women, but for her, they only added to Cal's attractiveness.

"Come on up here," Cathy said, waving Maya forward.

Maya nervously did as instructed, hoping her wobbly legs would survive the brief journey. Once the applause died down and Cathy announced that refreshments were about to served, Maya turned to the coconspirators.

"Can I have a word with both of you—privately, please?"

"Of course," Cathy said, exchanging a quick, wide-eyed glance with Cal. "But if this is about your name being called…you can thank Charlene for that. I told her you didn't want to be entered into the draw, and looks like she screwed up again."

Maya wasn't buying it for a second—especially after their strange behavior at the barn the other day. Now, it was all starting to make sense.

"Guys, I'm not dumb," she said, not sure whether to feel angry, annoyed…or maybe just a teensy-weensy bit thrilled that her earlier directive had been ignored.

"No...no you're not," Cal readily agreed, gazing into her eyes and dialing up the teensy-weensy by, oh, about a thousand notches.

Maya tried to stand her ground, not the easiest task when her roller-coaster feelings made her legs feel like spaghetti.

"Look, it's not the worst thing in the world—the two of us having dinner at a nice restaurant—is it?" Cal asked. "That's all this is."

Cathy tiptoed backward. "I think I just heard someone call my name. I'll catch up to you both later."

As she scurried off, Maya turned back to Cal. Their eyes once again met, but this time, they both slowly broke into a smile.

"That Charlene," Cal said with a feigned nonchalant shrug.

Maya grinned. "Yeah. That Charlene."

Okay, I think she's warming up to the idea, Cal thought as he gave silent thanks for the fact that she hadn't kicked in his kneecaps. In fact...if he didn't know any better, it *almost* looked like Maya wanted this dinner date as much as he did. And he wanted it a whole lot.

"So, I was looking online at restaurants the other night, and I came across one that's at the top of Mount Chester. Real cozy, with a couple of fireplaces in the dining room, and everything is cooked fresh from scratch."

Maya cocked her head to the side and flashed a half smirk. "Hmm. You went through a lot of trouble finding the perfect restaurant, considering you had no idea whose name would be called."

Cal knew she was one step short of calling his bluff, but he was more than happy to play along. "You know, that's just how I am. I'm a do-your-homework kind of guy."

"Huh. I didn't know that about you."

"Well, we'll have to use this dinner to get to know each other better."

As Maya's eyes widened, Cal cleared his throat and quickly added, "I mean, by talking. As colleagues. Nothing like good conversation to go with dinner."

Maya nodded, her deer-in-the-headlights visage slowly dropping away. "I agree."

I have my work cut out for me, Cal thought as he held on to the hope that the dinner would be the first course of Maya seeing him as more than a fellow vet.

And then what?

Even he couldn't answer that question. But the fact that he was asking it? That alone was nothing short of groundbreaking.

Maya entered her living room, dropping first her purse on the couch, and then herself. The fundraiser had wrapped up an hour ago, and after some friendly mingling with various townsfolk, she'd decided to make a quick getaway.

Everything seemed to be happening so fast, and she needed some time alone to think. Her cats Willow and Sam were quickly on her lap, and she laughed softly as they pawed at each other while competing for her attention. The rigid cast on her left arm made it more difficult to pet them both simultaneously, but she managed to improvise by bending her left elbow back as far as she could.

"I can't wait to get this thing off," she said, as much to herself as to the cats. She closed her eyes, silently acknowledging that her date night with Cal was another thing she couldn't wait for…but this realization was fraught with mixed feelings. The more she got attached to him, the harder it was going to be when he left Maplewood—and her life—for good. And the clock was already ticking on that end point.

A short time later, she quietly entered Jeremy's room, watching his blissfully peaceful face as he slept, illuminated by moonlight that shone through the side window.

Her smile wavered as she recalled standing in this very spot two years ago, slipping into the room to kiss Jeremy good night, only to be greeted by his tearful face. Even now, as she recalled the questions he had asked, there was a sharp tightness in her chest.

Why did Max leave? Did I do something wrong?

Maya drew in a breath with such force that she

feared the sound might wake her son. A few seconds passed, and relief set in as he continued to sleep.

She hated Max for breaking his heart. No—hate was too harmful of an emotion to hold onto. *I severely dislike what he did*, she revised in her thoughts. But still...some hate remained, only it was directed at herself, which somehow seemed more acceptable.

The truth was, Max had never made promises that he didn't keep. As their relationship evolved from strictly professional to also a romantic one, it had *seemed* like they were a family, just the three of them...but it was all an illusion. The word *forever* had never left his lips, so why had she assumed that's where things were headed?

She only knew one thing for certain at this point, which was that sometimes, the adage that "actions speak louder than words" was a load of bullcrap. Max had fully integrated himself into her and Jeremy's life like a husband and father, minus the official titles. And then, he was gone.

She couldn't—no, she *wouldn't*—make that mistake again.

The truth was, she could take care of herself. She'd had enough disappointment in recent years to know that if she were knocked down again, she'd manage to pick herself back up. Sure, she might get to the point of hanging a do-not-disturb sign off her heart, but she'd survive.

But Jeremy was still too young and vulnerable to

have the rug pulled out from under him again. Instinctively, Maya turned her gaze toward the dresser against the far side wall. In an almost mystical fashion, as if to say, *Look here*, a moonbeam had settled upon a framed picture of George holding a two-year-old Jeremy. George was smiling ear to ear, the proud father that he was, and Jeremy's eyes were half closed as he giggled during the shot.

Maya remembered taking that photo as though it were yesterday. It had always pained her to read how children didn't start forming memories until three years old—the exact age when Jeremy had lost his dad. Still, every once in a while, Jeremy would recall a specific moment with George, and she was grateful that he had those few but precious recollections.

But his memories with Max? There were many...

Maya shuddered as she tore herself away from her thoughts. It had been a long day, and certainly an eventful night. She leaned over and kissed Jeremy on the forehead, just soft enough to silently wish him a good night's sleep, but not enough to wake him.

It's just dinner with Cal...it doesn't mean anything, she said in her thoughts over and over again as she quietly closed Jeremy's bedroom door, then headed to the bathroom to wash up before bed. Staring through weary eyes at her reflection in the bathroom mirror, Maya knew one thing for sure. She was never good at lying—and that included to herself.

* * *

Sitting at the kitchen table after heading back from the fundraiser, Cal closed his laptop and breathed a sigh of relief. His reservation at White Peaks Restaurant was still booked for Saturday night. Not that he had any reason to think otherwise, but there was so much riding on this date that he needed to be sure.

There was so much riding on this date?

Even though the conclusion originated in his own brain, Cal still felt surprised by its implications. Was this actually going to be a date…as in a *date* date? Would Maya even allow as much?

He closed his eyes, picturing a small, intimate table by the fireplace, the flames casting a warm, sensual glow over Maya's exquisite face, her petite hand entwined in his…their lips about to touch…

Aruuuuu rooo rooo roo!

Cal popped an eye open. *Really? A coyote just destroyed my fantasy?*

He twisted his mouth to the side as several other coyotes joined the chorus. Was this the Vermont version of serenading a romantic interest? If so, he might as well make the most of it. With that, he closed his eyes again, picking up where he'd left off and brushing his lips against Maya's, pulling her in closer and feeling her petite body press against his…

"Hoo boy!" he exclaimed out loud, standing up abruptly from the chair. He tugged at the top of his shirt, feeling hot under the collar…and under the rest of his clothes, for that matter.

Sliding open the deck door, he took a pocket of chilled air into his lungs. Not exactly a cold shower, but it would do. "Woo!"

His exclamation started up another round of coyote howls, and pent-up angst gave way to laughter.

Stepping fully out onto the deck, Cal stared up at the starry sky, not allowing himself to dodge the second half of his earlier declaration.

A lot is riding on the date.

What did he mean by that? It was pretty bad when one had to question one's own statement…*but here we are*. He certainly had been on dates in the past with women he'd met during temporary vet gigs at one place or another, and it was never something he had felt the need to analyze ahead of time. Or during or after, for that matter.

But something was different with Maya. Was it because she'd made it clear that she had no intention of crossing the line from colleagues to something more?

He let that thought simmer for a moment, then realized it went beyond this. In the past, he knew that if he struck up a relationship with someone, it was bound to end once he moved on to the next gig. And he was okay with that. No—more like he *preferred* that scenario. But he wasn't feeling those "here today, gone tomorrow" vibes right now.

You'll feel that way when it's time to leave. That's just who you are.

Words that in some warped way would have comforted him in the past. But now, they felt oddly out of sync.

CHAPTER EIGHT

JAW JUTTED FORWARD and lips curled around her teeth, Maya stared into the bathroom mirror as she applied rose-colored lipstick. Smacking her lips, she admired the results for all of two seconds, her smile quickly turning into a frown.

She wiped the color off with a tissue, then glided her go-to clear, fruit-flavored lip gloss in its place, instantly satisfied with the swap.

Hey—at least I changed out of my jeans and stable boots, she thought as she looked down at her formfitting burgundy cocktail dress.

As she entered the kitchen a short time later, Carla looked up from the stove, where she was tending to a sizzling stir-fry.

"I shouldn't be too late," Maya said, leaving out the unspoken addendum of *unless Cal kisses me, in which case, I won't be in a rush to come home.*

She nearly shuddered at her own thoughts.

Don't go there. Don't go there. Don't go there.

Carla smiled at her—almost a little too knowingly, Maya surmised.

"That's fine. Jeremy and I have a fun night planned. After dinner, we're going to watch the latest Marvel movie, and I've got some popcorn and cocoa lined up for when the munchies strike."

Maya smiled. "That sounds great." She paused, looking out into the living room that opened from the kitchen. "Speaking of my little guy...where is he?"

"He's out playing with Rusty."

As if on cue, the front door at the far end of the living room flew open, and Jeremy and Rusty bounded inside.

"Look at you!" Maya said affectionately as Jeremy breathlessly made his way over, dirt caked on his cheek. Maya cocked her head to the side as she spotted a matching dirt patch on Rusty's nose. "Did you guys get in a mud-wrestling match?"

"We were running and I tripped, and Rusty was trying to nudge me up from the ground."

Maya petted the loyal golden retriever, who was now by her side. "What a good boy," she said affectionately. Rusty looked up at her with wide amber eyes, tongue hanging out in a rapid pant.

"Are you leaving for your date with Cal?" Jeremy asked matter-of-factly.

Maya's hand froze in midstroke of Rusty's silky fur. She swallowed down a gulp, and then another one. "It's not... I'm not..." Now *she* was the one sporting wide eyes with a nervous pant. "It's a fundraiser thing for Happy Hooves, that's all. Cal wanted to help the horses like Molly by being a participant, and my name was called in the draw. Just a...a weird coincidence."

Maya glanced over at Carla, who quickly diverted her gaze back to the stir-fry, a widening smirk on her face.

Great. Even Carla suspects something's up.

Jeremy shrugged, then looked down at Rusty. "Come on, I'll feed you now."

As the two trotted off, indifferent to the date-or-no-date debate, Maya laughed and shook her head. Spotting headlights closing in on the picture window facing the driveway, Maya caught her breath. Cal had arrived, and there was no turning back now. And what troubled her even more? She didn't *want* to turn back. *Uh-uh. Nope.*

"Enjoy your non-date," Carla said with a barely suppressed grin as Maya headed out the door.

"*Carla...*" Maya tried to sound ominous, but her pretend warning only made Carla's grin widen.

Cal pulled Maya's chair out at the restaurant and waited for her to be seated before pushing the chair back in. At least that was the plan, but his hands grabbed onto air as she scooted it back to the table herself. *We've got to work on this roll-out-the-red-carpet thing*, he surmised with a tinge of amusement, recalling how she similarly had hopped into his truck earlier in the evening before he'd had a chance to open the door for her.

When drinks arrived at the table ten minutes later, Cal raised his glass of beer. "To Happy Hooves."

Maya repeated the toast with a clink of her wineglass.

"So am I allowed to tell you that you look beautiful tonight?"

Maya blushed while simultaneously looking pleased by the compliment. "Thank you." She held up her cast. "I was worried about a color clash, but what the heck. Burgundy and turquoise are the new orange and black."

Her smile prompted a small crinkle on the side of her left eye that Cal found endearing. *No*—sexily *endearing*, he silently revised.

After the waiter came by to take their order, Cal took in his surroundings. It was hard to look away from Maya, but as her eyes scanned the dining room, he decided to do the same.

"This place is amazing," he said, nodding appreciatively at the warmly lit string lights, two roaring fireplaces, aromatic pumpkin candles and autumn-themed pine wreaths scattered about. "Have you been here before?"

"A few times."

Maya's reply was terser than Cal expected, and though he was curious to know more, he decided not to pry. He didn't have to.

"The last time I was here was with Max." Running her finger over the rim of her wineglass, Maya paused, as though debating whether to say more.

"He was a vet at Northern Vermont Equine Associates, and we ended up in a relationship that lasted nearly two years. Another horse vet. I guess you could say I have a type."

Okay, now we're getting somewhere. He waited for her to elaborate, but was met with silence.

"So...did he leave the practice because the relationship ended?" he gently nudged.

"More like the other way around. I thought things were serious with us—enough so that I'd be a part of any major life decisions. Instead, he announced out of the blue one day that he'd been offered a position at a practice out in Texas. It was affiliated with a major university, so he'd have a prestigious teaching role as well. I mean, I did understand the allure of the position."

"Did he ask if you wanted to join him?"

"No, but in his defense, he already knew the answer. My home is here—and my work. Not that I couldn't leave my current practice for another. People change jobs all the time." She paused to flash a wry grin. "Not that I need to tell someone like *you* that."

"Ouch." Cal felt the pinch of that pointed poke... and liked it. He'd take a woman who spoke her mind any day over one who played "guess what I'm thinking" games as a side hobby.

"Anyway, point being, my dad built the practice from the ground up, and I couldn't imagine tossing it all aside to go chase after someone else's dream.

My dream is here, the town I grew up in, where I'm raising my son and I still have family, and clients that I love. I know this probably sounds way too provincial for some people, and I get it. But this is what makes me happy."

Cal nodded, his eyes still focused intently on Maya. Everything that she had just said made sense. She was happy here. She loved her job and was surrounded by family. But...was it just him who felt there was something missing from this equation? *Such as...oh, I don't know...a partner? Someone to share it with.*

Maya stared back at him with widening eyes. "What?" To *his* widened eyes, she added, "You look like you want to say something."

"Only that I can understand why you wouldn't want to leave here."

Maya silently assessed him, as though not entirely buying that he *could* understand her priorities.

"The worst part of Max's leaving was how it affected Jeremy," she said pensively.

Cal took a deep breath and leaned back in his chair. He obviously didn't know Max, not that he could possibly learn anything additional about the man that would raise him up from the depths of Loserville. But the fact that his actions hurt Jeremy? Yeah...that was an unforgivable offense.

"In some ways, it was harder on him losing Max than his own father," Maya continued, "but only because he was so young when George died. I always wonder what would have happened if I hadn't let him take my place for the emergency call. Would Jeremy still have both parents? Or..."

He knew what she was thinking, even though it remained unsaid: Would Jeremy have lost her to a drunk driver instead?

"But, I'll never know because he *did* take my place."

Cal could almost viscerally feel the undeserved guilt over his death that he knew she'd been carrying around for years. "That's what good husbands do," he said quietly.

Maya seemed surprised by his comment. Maybe she didn't think he was capable of knowing what made a decent husband. *Fair enough.*

"When you showed up at the barn for Buttercup's emergency, it reminded me of George." Maya silently gasped, then gave a quick headshake. "I'm sorry—that didn't come out quite right."

"It's okay. I know what you're trying to say." *Kind of, sort of...*

"I'm glad, because you're two very different people in other ways."

In mid-lift of his beer glass, Cal paused, then decided to take a sip so as not to appear too taken aback. Still...*what did she mean by that?*

"You mean because I'm Australian?" he asked, unable to fully let go of the comment.

Maya seemed caught off guard by the question. "No, more like George loved his home and his family. He didn't have your adventurous spirit. That's all I meant."

"Oh." Cal was unsure how to feel about this observation, but he understood how she'd naturally arrived there. After all, how could he come across as anything but the antithesis of a dedicated family man, given that he'd never been able to stick around long enough for a permanent job or a place to put down roots?

Tearing away from his thoughts, Cal once again looked into Maya's eyes. She held his gaze, and he felt an unspoken understanding pass between them. He wondered if she was thinking what he was…and hoped this wasn't the case. Or was it best that she did? Because the last thing he'd ever want to do was hurt her, and right now, in his sea of thoughts, there was one that kept bobbing to the surface.

I am so *not the kind of man that she wants or needs.*

He was grateful when their meals arrived a short time later. Truth be told, his appetite had taken a hit as the conversation had veered toward conclusions—or one in particular—that left a bitter taste in his mouth. But at least with a plate of clam linguini in front of him, he could keep his mouth occupied with something other than his foot.

"So," Maya began, throwing a wrench, or more like a fork, in his plans to stay mum. "You did say this dinner was a chance to get to know each other better. I've had my turn on the confessional—now it's yours."

"I said that?"

A one-sided grin. "You did."

Cal squelched a grimace as his words came back to bite him in the butt. *Again.*

Still, he managed to actually sound almost gregarious in his reply. "There's nothing to say. My life has been boring."

Maya nearly spit out a sip of wine. "Says the guy who's lived all over the world and probably has a gal stashed away at every port."

Now it was Cal's turn to choke on his drink. "Uh...no, that's definitely not the case."

Maya playfully cocked her head to the side. "At every train station?"

Cal chuckled, partly out of amusement and partly to avoid having to explain his life choices. How could he *not* come across as an untethered stallion, galloping from one field or tundra to another, no mare deemed special enough to rein him in?

He inwardly rolled his eyes at himself. *Hey, you're a horse guy—what else are you going to use for an analogy? Cars?*

But Maya wasn't finished. "Come on. I thought we were going to be real with each other tonight. Not to mention that I spent three hundred dollars on Hunks for Horses tickets—including the one responsible for us being here right now." She paused, adding mischievously, "You know—because *Charlene* accidentally added it to the bucket."

"Okay, you're right," Cal finally acquiesced with a chuckle. "What do you want to know?"

Maya shrugged her slender shoulders, in more of a flirty than indifferent manner. "What makes Cal tick?"

A simple question, and yet Cal was stumped. In part because no one had ever asked him this before. And certainly not someone who'd captured his full attention like Maya had.

Should he cherry-pick what to tell her, given that there were far more sour than sweet cherries in his background? He pondered the question for a moment. He rarely shared much of his past with others. No—that wasn't quite accurate. He *never* did, and that included with women he'd dated in the past.

Not that some of them hadn't probed him to learn more. But what was the point of sharing such personal details with them? Better that they knew him as the life of the party, rather than a killjoy whose past could suck all the happiness out of a room.

But with Maya, something was different. She had a grounded, drama-free air about her that made him feel safe to open up. *Feel safe to open up?* Cal bristled at the thought. Now was not the time to psychoanalyze why he'd been a closed book with other people in his life, and now with Maya, he was ready to turn the page. Or at least skim through a foreword that touched upon his past.

The drug-addicted mother who had abandoned him at birth. The father he had never known. The string of foster homes where genuine love and care had been in short, if any, supply. And the one exception to all of this—his time on the horse ranch with Thomas and Mabel and a life-altering bond with a timid mustang named Flaxxie that had started out hopeful, but ultimately led to heartache.

When he finished, Maya stared at him in stunned silence. "Cal, that's just…" She paused, clearly still grappling with his unexpected revelations. "I had no idea."

"Not many people do," Cal said, a slight fib given it implied that at least a *few* other people were privy to his past. But that was a few more than the actual reality.

"I'm trying to think of what my life would be like if I hadn't had family like I do…and my brain simply can't go there. I can't imagine what it must be like not to feel that someone's looking out for you, no matter what." She paused, her face pained.

There was no way Cal was going to let *his* life circumstances bring Maya down. Which meant he needed to put a positive spin on things…and fast.

"You have nothing to be sorry for. In some ways, it's been my superpower."

Maya blinked hard with surprise. "What do you mean?"

"Don't get me wrong—I'm sure it's great to have the support system of a solid family, but not having that has its benefits, too. The decisions I make—the jobs I take, the places I live—are based on where I think I can make the biggest difference. I don't have to confer with anyone else before making a move. I can just do it."

Maya started to open her mouth as if to speak, then stopped.

Cal cocked his head slightly to the side. "Go ahead—you were going to say something."

"You're right. I was going to say that sounds lonely, but then I realized I was projecting my own feelings about things onto you. Like I said—you have an adventurous spirit. So why be tied down by anything...or anyone. Right?"

Coming from anyone else, this observation would have sounded like a thinly veiled insult. But Cal knew that Maya was genuinely trying to understand what motivated him in life. He'd avoided sharing such personal revelations over the years and now he knew why. No one would've had the capacity—or desire—to truly empathize with his past actions and decisions like Maya was demonstrating now.

"And I would imagine the situation with Molly has brought up a lot of painful memories for you," Maya said quietly.

Cal pursed his lips and nodded. "There's been a few times that I actually caught myself thinking that Molly is Flaxxie, which I know sounds crazy."

"It doesn't," Maya said gently. "You didn't have the happy ending that you should have had with

Flaxxie, and it's going to mean that much more when Molly pulls through."

Cal wondered if Maya truly believed that Molly was on the road to a certain recovery, or if she was piling on the hope for all of their sakes—but especially his.

"So, what was it about coming here that drew you in?" Maya asked after a span of silence ensured. "And I mean to Vermont, and Northern Vermont Equine Associates."

"Well, I'd never been to New England before, and there were actually a few opportunities that I was looking into. But then I talked to your dad, and that really sealed the deal for me."

A slight smile formed on Maya's lips. "How so?"

"He talked about you, and how you were trying to almost single-handedly keep the practice running, despite having a broken arm and cracked ribs. I almost couldn't believe what I was hearing, to be honest. It's hard enough doing this job with no broken bones, never mind *with*."

Maya grinned. "No argument there."

"Plus, just hearing the worry and concern in his voice when he talked about you. That's the kind of dad that everyone should have, and I felt I could really help out in this situation."

Maya met his eyes and held his gaze. He felt a tingling warmth travel the length of his body, and it wasn't from the pepper sauce on his green bean salad.

"I'm glad my dad didn't listen to me when I told him not to hire you."

Cal did a double take. Or maybe it was triple. "Seriously?"

Maya briefly chuckled at his reaction. "Don't take it personally. I hadn't met you yet, and let's just say I was a little apprehensive about having a new colleague encroach on my territory."

Cal raised an amused eyebrow. "Sounds like you've been picking up some alpha mare behaviors."

"Ha! You might be right about that."

Walking out to the parking lot forty minutes later after a shared dessert of maple-infused cheesecake, cognac-spiked coffee and more easy conversation borne out of their natural rapport, Cal stopped short of his truck and turned to Maya.

"So apparently there's a lookout tower at the very top of this mountain that's open twenty-four seven. It's a short drive from here. I thought maybe we could do some stargazing after this? It has a glass elevator, so you don't have to worry about climbing stairs in those four-inch heels."

Maya smiled nervously. "Three-inch heels," she said after a long pause. Though something told Cal her delayed answer had little to do with footwear aesthetics.

Maya let Cal's question float in the air as she tried to get her bearings. She'd been enjoying this night with Cal so much that she almost forgot a few hard truths behind it. Beginning with the fact that Monday morning, at exactly 8:00 a.m., she and Cal would be showing up at the clinic together, ready to start another day as colleagues.

Repeat after me. AS COLLEAGUES.

And what happened when colleagues became romantically involved? She grimaced at her own question. *Nothing good, I can tell you that.*

Still, despite her small inner voice that was seemingly being filtered through a megaphone, she felt compelled to dig into this some more.

What was the worst that could happen if—just this once—she approached things like Cal? Which meant fully realizing from the get-go that the situation between them was temporary. No hand-wringing about what would happen when he left, which was inevitable. No getting attached. Simply living in the moment, and when the moment ended, so did all the feelings.

Could she even do this? It was such a departure from who she was at her core. But maybe that's why she *needed* to switch things up, to get out of her comfort zone and peel back a layer of the protective shell that surrounded her.

And then…an image of Jeremy flashed in her mind. Because none of this was just about her. Far from it. Nor did she have to question whose needs mattered most—hers or her son's. Hands down, she had to do what was best for him. Case unequivocally closed.

She looked back at Cal, a pang in her side as she mentally prepared to shoot down his invitation. "I think I should call it a night. I told Jeremy I wouldn't be out late and..." Her voice trailed off.

Cal rolled his lips together as though trying to smile, but not quite getting there. "Of course. I understand."

Maya wondered if he actually did grasp her inner dilemma, but either way, he seemed to respect her decision. And she really couldn't ask for more than that.

As they resumed walking farther out into the parking lot, Cal looked up at the sky and pointed to a long purple nebula intertwined with streaks of light and stars.

"Wow—look at that."

Maya glanced upward. "The Milky Way. Amazing."

"Who needs an observation tower, I guess."

"Right?" Maya wondered if her one-word reply sounded as awkward as it felt.

Dropping her gaze from the sky, she looked back at Cal, trying to stay fully in the moment. But the moment was inextricably tied to the past. *Cal's* past. He had revealed things to her that she never would have imagined. Things that happened to him in his youth that could have turned him into a hard and bitter adult. He had neither of these qualities...but only because he'd chosen a path of self-reliance and spurned attachments of any kind. Could she blame him?

Staring into his eyes, she voiced the answer in her mind. *No.* A realization that only further cemented the need to avoid any attachment herself. And kissing him was not going to further that agenda. Not with the off-the-charts desire that was coursing through her body.

Change the subject. Look back up at the sky. Remove your lips from the scene—STAT!

Of course, Cal couldn't hear any of the hurried directives playing out in her mind. A good thing, given that he was apparently on course to kiss her lips, and nothing was holding him back.

He pulled her close, running his fingers through the back of her hair, pressing his hard, muscular chest against hers, kissing her lips slowly at first, and then more hungrily. She met his rhythm, then took it up a notch. He responded to her eagerness by pulling her closer, if that was even possible.

Her body went limp, and she began to teeter on heels with legs that were far more used to stable boots. Sensing her unsteadiness, Cal picked up the slack...or more precisely, picked up *her*. Feet dangling several inches off the ground, their lips continued their dance, pulling away, brushing close, reengaging, again and again.

When Maya's feet touched the ground in what seemed like an eternity later, she could only manage to utter one word. "Wow."

Cal slowly grinned. "I second that."

"Ouch!" She leaned forward and grabbed her side as a sharp pain took hold.

"What's wrong? Are you okay?"

She drew in a deep breath. "Yes—strange. It's like I had a delayed reaction to my ribs being squeezed." Seeing the concern on his face, she quickly added, "Don't worry—I'm fine." A tentative pause, and then a smile. "It was worth a few seconds of fleeting rib pain."

As Cal's face softened, she wondered if it was a good idea to be indirectly encouraging more of the same. The uncrossable line had been crossed, and it was potentially a quick, straight path to go from a single kiss to so much more. But that didn't mean it was a journey she should take.

Looking back up at Cal, Maya saw anything but caution in Cal's eyes. *But he's not the one who's in danger of having his heart broken.* So she'd have to be the one to drive what happens next.

"Well, I most certainly got my money's worth with this...outing...tonight," she said softly, the word *date* unable to launch from her lips. Not after everything that had just played out in her mind.

Cal dipped his head slightly to the side, studying her through slightly squinted eyes as he sized up her words.

She should have known he'd be perceptive enough to pick up on what other men would've missed.

"Glad you enjoyed yourself," he said, reaching

over to open the passenger door. "And at least this time, I can help you into the truck."

Maya smiled, but as he took her hand to boost her up into the raised seat, she looked away.

Don't let him see your eyes, she told herself. Because if it were true that eyes were windows to the soul, then he'd see how much she wished that circumstances could be otherwise.

CHAPTER NINE

THE ANXIOUS CALL from Cathy came late in the afternoon, not long after Maya and Cal had returned from a shared visit to a large horse farm several towns over for routine exams. What had initially seemed like a promising start to a near-certain recovery for Molly had begun to whittle away with day-by-day setbacks, and now with another seizure, she had taken a sharp turn for the worse.

Maya called over to Jeremy, who'd been dropped off earlier after school by Gus so he could accompany them for a recheck on Molly. But that was before she'd received the grave news.

"Jeremy, I think it's best that you stay here. Maria can watch you until Grandpa can pick you up. It doesn't sound good for Molly, and we might have to make a very difficult decision."

"I still want to see her," he said, his eyes glossy as he struggled to hold back tears.

Feeling another set of eyes upon her, Maya looked over at Cal. He was watching them both intently, and as his gaze locked on to hers, she knew he disagreed with the decision she'd just made.

I'm the parent, she wanted to say. But perhaps that was the crux of the problem. She was trying to protect Jeremy in the event that Molly would have to be euthanized. Even when it was done in the horse's best interest, when there were no other options and it was a means to end suffering, it was still a heart-wrenching task. This was true even for a very senior horse who had lived out a full and comfortable life up until the point when their body began to give out. But for a young horse in her prime like Molly? *You'll get used to it*, she'd been told in vet school. That was fifteen years ago...and there were still times that she'd hold in her tears just long enough to complete the end-of-life procedure, waiting until she was back in her truck before allowing the dam to break.

Maya turned back to Jeremy, weighing the pros and cons of allowing him to accompany her and Cal—and weighing them fast, knowing the clock was ticking. If they did have to put Molly down, he'd have a chance to say goodbye. That didn't mean he had to witness her final moments—they could figure all that out once they assessed the situation.

She reached over and squeezed his arm. "Okay, why don't you get in the truck, and Cal and I will join you in a second."

"I hope I'm doing the right thing," Maya said quietly as Cal came up to her side.

"I think you are. I know how difficult this is, but closure is just as important for kids as it is for us adults."

"I just keep hoping we'll discover something that

we missed earlier…something that could turn things around."

"Me too. And we don't know yet that nothing can be done." He nodded to the truck. "Let's go see if we can pull off a miracle."

As Maya entered Molly's stall after a white-knuckle drive to the rescue, she knew that a miracle was probably not going to happen.

"I think that last seizure took everything she had," Cathy said quietly, her voice choking up as they all peered down at Molly, who was lying on her side, only the faintest rise in her chest indicating that she was still alive.

As Cal placed a comforting hand on Maya's shoulder, she briefly closed her eyes and placed her hand on top of it. So many times in the course of her career, she'd had to make the most difficult decisions and be privy to the most heartbreaking scenes alone. But as their hands touched, she felt buoyed by Cal's strength—not just his physicality, but his emotional depth as well. Everyone in that stall right now was hurting badly over what had to be done, and he was right there in the thick of it with them.

"Is there anything else we can do?" Cathy asked, her face gaunt and pale.

"We've tried all the medications," Cal said, "She's just not responding to them in a way that most horses would."

Maya knew that there was always a subset of horses with EPM that continued to go downhill after commencing treatment. That Molly would be one of them was a fate too cruel for words.

"I don't want her to suffer anymore," Cathy said, no longer able to hold back tears.

Maya nodded, the professional in her putting a stoic face forward, the mother and horse lover in her inwardly struggling to maintain her composure.

She walked over to Jeremy and gently grasped both of his small hands. "Jeremy..."

She swallowed several times, struggling to say the words.

"You have to put Molly down," he said solemnly, saying them for her.

"Yes. We don't want her to suffer anymore. Do you want to say goodbye to her?"

As he wiped tears from his eyes, Maya felt like she'd been pummeled in the gut by a pair of unseen fists.

She held his hand as they walked over to Molly, then let go as he dropped to his knees beside her head.

"I love you, Molly," he said, leaning over and stroking her mane. "I'm so sorry this happened to you."

The sight was almost more than Maya could bear. She turned to Cal, his eyes as pained as hers as he watched the scene play out.

An eerie silence filled the stall, pierced at intervals by Jeremy's muffled sobs. Maya gently clasped his shoulders and turned him toward her.

"Honey, you don't have to stay for this. You said goodbye to Molly, and I know she heard you. You can wait in the truck—"

"I want to stay."

Maya nodded, the lump in her throat now the size of a hard plum. "Okay, why don't you go over and stand with Cathy."

As he joined Cathy against the left-facing stall wall, she wrapped her arm tightly around his side.

Cal was already placing the catheter in Molly's jugular vein when Maya turned her attention back to the mare. She pulled her vet bag over and took out a vial of detomidine, a sedative typically administered to calm a horse before the fatal dose of pentobarbital.

"Just in case," she said in a low voice between them. Though Molly was already fully subdued, the last thing she wanted was for her to suddenly begin to stir and then fight the effects of the pentobarbital. Not only did she not want this to define Molly's last moments, but she'd do anything to spare Jeremy from witnessing such a distressing sight.

Cal nodded in agreement, leaning back to give Maya room to inject the sedative into the catheter. She waited several moments, then prepared to administer a bolus of pentobarbital. Drawing 300 milligrams into the syringe, she momentarily closed her eyes, drawing on her dwindling reserves of willpower in order to carry out what needed to be done.

"Wait."

Maya's eyes sprung open with Cal's one-word directive. She followed his line of vision to where Jeremy stood, wiping his eyes with his sleeve as Cathy pulled him in even tighter.

"Cal..." she said quietly, her own heart aching beyond words. For Molly, for her son...

But she couldn't let Molly suffer any longer. Taking a deep breath, she positioned the needle to insert into the catheter. One push of the plunger, and Molly's suffering would end. This young, beautiful mare who had already been through so much in her short lifetime.

Maya stared at the plunger as time stood still. She could hear Jeremy's faint sniffles, like a stab in the heart. Had she made the right decision by letting him stay through the procedure?

Her hand, normally so steady in the direst of medical circumstances, shook slightly as she gripped the syringe.

You have no choice.

Doubling down to focus through tear-filled eyes, Maya placed her thumb against the plunger as she readied to expel its contents.

"I said wait!" Cal exclaimed.

This time, there was a flash of anger in Maya's eyes as she glared up at Cal. Why was he making this infinitely more difficult than it already was? He knew as well as she did that they had no choice but to carry out this devastating but necessary decision.

"There might be another way."

Maya didn't understand. "To euthanize her?"
"To save her."
As Cathy let out an audible gasp, Maya's breath caught in her throat. She glanced back at Jeremy, wondering why Cal would give her son false hope like this. *He should know better.*

"We know the medication was doing its job killing the parasite," Cal said, taking a step closer.

"And sometimes that's not enough." Maya's voice nearly cracked as she tried to hold everything together. "I've seen this before in severe EPM cases. It's the neurological damage that's left behind—that's what does these horses in."

She stroked Molly's flaxen mane, her unmoving yet still-pristine body making this moment feel all the more unfathomable. None of it made sense—not on a philosophical level, the age-old question of why life was sometimes so cruel. But it made sense from a veterinary medicine standpoint, as much as she wished it hadn't.

"I know," Cal said, his voice subdued yet strong at the same time. He kneeled down beside Molly and rested his hand on her neck, scanning the length of her with a sadness in his eyes. "But what if we could address the neurological issues?"

"We can't," Maya replied, more sharply than she intended. "I mean, we already tried that."

"With the usual drugs—yes. But what about something experimental? We've got nothing to lose at this point."

"Cal—we're out of time. We don't have months or years to wait for a drug to be developed that could change anything." She stared hard into his eyes. He *had* to know this. Why in the world was he tossing out crazy ideas?

"I know. But a drug already exists. Before my last gig in California, I worked for a few months at a large practice in Ohio. One of the vets also worked in research at a local agricultural university. They developed a drug—dorfamin—that repaired neurological damage in clinical trials."

Maya's heart skipped a beat. "For horses?"

"For cows. They were trying to find a cure for mad cow disease."

Maya's shoulders dropped. It wasn't the answer she hoped to hear, but Cal clearly didn't share her skepticism.

"I read through all the white papers and clinical data. It's legit, Maya. I won't go into the details—there's no time—but the mechanism of how the drug worked to reverse neurological damage in cows would theoretically be the same for horses."

"Is this drug available locally?"

"No," Cal said, his eyes darting to the side, as though he was searching for a viable solution. "It's still experimental and not on the market. That's why I didn't even think of it earlier." He pulled his phone out of the front pocket of his jeans and scrolled through the screen. "I still have Joe's number." He looked up, meeting Maya's eyes, then glanced over at Jeremy. Turning back to Maya, he said, "Let me go call him now."

She nodded, almost too numb by the sudden turn of events to react further.

"What's going on?" Cathy asked as Cal exited the stall to talk privately in the barn aisle.

Maya pulled her off to the side and quietly filled her in. Cathy's mouth was still agape as Cal reentered the stall.

"Okay," he said, pausing to take a deep breath.

It took great restraint for Maya not to shout, *What did you find out?*

"The drug still isn't on the market yet, but the patent was bought by a pharmaceutical company for further development."

"So it's not available?" Cathy asked, echoing Maya's silent conclusion.

"Joe said he has an in with the drugmaker and can get us enough medication for a full course of treatment. But it will cost five thousand dollars. He said there's no way around that, now that they officially own the patent."

Cathy shook her head with disgust. "Typical pharmaceutical company price gouging. Bastards." She shook her head again, then looked back up at Maya and Cal. "I don't have that kind of money. Between stocking up on enough hay for winter, and paying a contractor to put a new roof on the second barn, all the fundraiser money has already been spent.

And even if I ran another fundraiser just for this, I wouldn't be able to raise the full amount in time."

She looked down at Molly's seemingly lifeless body, her breath so slow and shallow that it escaped limited human perception. "I'm not a vet obviously, but she would need to be treated, like...*now*."

"I have the money," Cal said, as Maya jerked her head up. There was a collective gasp as Maya and Cathy reacted to Cal's shocking announcement.

"Cal! You can't..." Maya's voice dropped off.

"Can't what?" he asked with quiet forcefulness. "Spend my money on what I want? *This* is what I want."

"Wait." Maya's head was beyond spinning as she tried to piece together the logistics of making a potential miracle happen. "Even if you pay for it, I don't see how we'd get it in time."

"It's an hour's plane ride to Ohio."

Maya's mouth dropped open. Whatever the word was for *crazy times ten*...that's where this situation had landed. She drew in a deep breath, knowing she needed to stay calm and collected—not the easiest of feats under the circumstances.

"The airport is an hour away. And I'm not trying to be a Negative Nelly here, but the chances of there being a direct flight to Ohio today are pretty slim." She looked down at Molly, not wanting to lose sight of what truly was at stake. Her life. The chance for survival, which, only several minutes ago, was nonexistent. Maybe it was still too much to hope for...

"There's a small local airport twenty minutes from here," Cal said, cutting into her thoughts. "I know because I looked into it when I decided to take this job. I have a pilot's license, and they rent out single-engine planes."

It took a moment for Maya to reply as she tried to wrap her head around yet another *where did this come from?* revelation.

"Is there something else I should know about you?" she asked, dumbfounded. "Are you also a secret intelligence agent in your spare time?"

Cal revealed the hint of a smile, which, given the gravity of the situation, was the most that anyone could muster in the moment. "Joe said there's a landing strip in one of the fields at the university. They use it to fly in agricultural supplies. He'll meet us there with the medication. If we leave now, we can be back here in a few hours." He paused. "There's just one thing."

"What?" Maya asked.

"Given that I'm here on a work visa, it's possible there'll be some red tape to cut through before they allow me to rent a plane. I mean…maybe not, but I don't want to take any chances. If one of you comes with me, it could help move things along."

"I'll go," Cathy offered. She turned to Maya. "That way, you can keep an eye on Molly. I wouldn't know what to do if things take a turn for the worse."

Maya wasn't sure how things could possibly get more critical for Molly, but she understood where

Cathy was coming from. Still, without the medication, all hope was lost—so securing it needed to be the top priority now.

"Thanks, Cathy. But I think I should go—only because I can show my practice credentials and that might give us an edge if there's an issue." She paused, directing her gaze at Cathy and then Cal. "Hopefully, there's a horse lover or two working at the airport today."

Cal pulled his lips together in a tight smile as he nodded.

"What about Molly?" Cathy asked, her voice shaky with a mix of worry and optimistic excitement.

Maya pulled her phone out of her jacket pocket, scrolled to her father's number and waited several rings for the call to be answered.

"Hey, Maya—"

"Dad, how soon can you get to Happy Hooves?" she hurriedly interjected.

"I can leave now." There was a several-second pause before he asked, "Is everything okay?"

"Yes…sort of. It's kind of a long story, but Cathy will fill you in when you get here. Jeremy's here, too."

A quick thank-you and goodbye, and then Maya turned to Cathy. "My dad will know what to do once you give him the background of what's going on. We don't want to oversedate Molly, so once it starts to wear off, he'll need to monitor her and keep her safe until we get back."

Jeremy...

In the midst of one new development bubbling up after another, Maya's attention had unintentionally been diverted from her son. A pang of guilt gripped her as she hurried over to him and wrapped him in a tight hug. "Grandpa's going to be here soon."

"Can you and Cal save Molly?"

Another grab at her gut, this one provoked by the possibility that she was only prolonging an inevitable sad ending.

"We're going to try. But Jeremy, Molly is very, very sick, and the drug we're going to get might not be enough to turn things around. But Cal thinks there's a possibility it could work, so we want to give her that chance."

He nodded, understanding emanating from his light gray eyes. Maybe he was more attuned to the oftentimes fast-shifting realities of life than she gave him credit for.

"I love you," she said, leaning in and kissing him on the forehead. His hair smelled fruity, and she smiled at the realization that he had been using her shampoo again, rather than his own ocean-breeze soap-and-shampoo combo, made especially for kids. Not that she could blame him. Who didn't want to smell like fresh strawberries?

"I love you, too."

She stood up and turned to Cal. "Ready?"

He nodded, opening the stall gate to leave, then abruptly turning around. As he went to kneel by Molly, running his hand across her side, Maya joined him.

"She looks so beautiful and peaceful," she said quietly. "It's hard to believe..."

As Cal reached over and placed his hand over hers, Maya's breath caught in her throat. She felt his strength run through her. Strength of conviction. Strength of hope. And just plain...*strength*. That of the physical kind, a solid warmth that enveloped her entire hand. And suddenly, in this make-or-break moment with Molly's life hanging in the balance and so much on the line...she felt she could handle whatever the outcome would be. They'd celebrate a miracle together—her hope against hope—or they'd lean on each other to get through the heartbreak.

As a thought entered her head that she might be expecting more from Cal than he could give, she pushed it away. *Not now.* And when that thought returned, as it inevitably would? She'd deal with it then.

Cal radioed into Vermont's North Central Airport, advising the control tower that headwinds had put him fifteen minutes ahead of schedule.

Just over three hours had passed since he and Maya had left—or more like raced—from Happy Hooves Horse Rescue, and it had been the fastest, and yet longest, three hours of his life.

So far, everything had gone according to plan—a miracle in itself given that the plan had been whipped up last minute, or more precisely, last second. With Maya by his side, they had breezed through the plane rental logistics, careening down the grassy landing strip at the University of Ohio one hour and eighteen minutes later.

Joe and several of his medical research team were waiting for them, and after a quick exchange and instructions, Cal and Maya were once again looking over the clouds.

He turned to her now, greeted by her long, dark ash-brown hair as she faced the side window. Silence had filled the cockpit for most of the departing flight, and now that they were three-quarters of the way back, he was itching the break the impasse.

"You're being very quiet."

She turned to him and forced a smile. "I'm just enjoying the scenery."

He raised an eyebrow. "You mean the cloud cover?" Which was more or less his way of saying, *Um...no, you're not.*

He waited for her to reply, and then waited some more. "I know you're worried that I'm giving Jeremy false hope."

Maya turned to him again, and this time her eyes flashed with emotion. Whether it was anger or worry, he couldn't tell. Maybe it was a bit of both. "*Are* you giving him false hope?" she asked, her voice quiet yet sharp at the same time.

Cal closed his eyes for a moment, wondering how to answer her question. Not because he was trying to sugarcoat reality, but because there was no way he could definitively answer that question. No one could.

"I can't say for certain that this drug will save Molly. When it comes to medicine, nothing is foolproof, whether it's experimental or a staple that's been around for fifty years. But I wouldn't have suggested this treatment if I didn't think it could possibly work."

He quietly sighed, knowing that his answer, though truthful, didn't directly address Maya's question. If only he could express the depths of his own emotions right now, he thought. But it was a chasm so deep that he wouldn't even know where to start.

"I saw you look at Jeremy right before I was about to administer the pentobarbital. Would you have suggested this experimental option if he hadn't been there?"

Cal took in a deep breath. "I don't know." He turned to her again, searching her eyes. "To be honest, I'm not sure if trying this other drug would've even occurred to me. Like I said, it's not on the market and it wasn't developed specifically for horses. But then I saw Jeremy crying…and it took me back to being that boy myself. I knew what he was feeling in that moment, thinking that Molly wasn't going to make it. The same, most horrible feeling that I had when Flaxxie disappeared and I wasn't able to find her. I know not all kids get attached to animals like I did, but I see that same quality in Jeremy. And I was thinking in that moment, I would do anything—*anything*—to save Molly's life, and to spare him that pain." He paused, his eyes boring into hers. "And to spare *you* that pain as his mother. And that's when this other drug suddenly popped into my head."

She held his gaze for several moments, then pursed her lips and nodded slightly. "Jeremy's a lot like me in how he naturally bonds to animals. I was the same way as a kid. I think I had more animal friends than human ones. Something tells me you might have been the same."

"For sure."

"I'm still like that, actually. It's easy to trust animals, to know their love is pure and unconditional. It's not always that way with people." Maya paused, as though briefly reliving some of the disappointments that had fueled this conclusion, then looked back at Cal. "But I'd say you're about as close to a horse in my eyes as a human can get."

Cal's breath caught in his throat, but as Maya slowly began to smile, he felt the mood lighten. "I don't think I've ever been paid a higher compliment," he said with a grin. And he meant it.

Still, he could see the effort behind Maya's smile, the anxiousness that hadn't left her eyes. He reached over and clasped her small hand. It tensed up in a ball underneath his grasp, then slowly relaxed.

"It's going to be okay, Maya," he said quietly, ignoring the small inner voice that warned him not to make promises he couldn't keep.

"I don't know the ins and outs of this treatment like you do, but I do know it might not work."

Cal felt his insides plummet, as though the plane had just taken a nosedive. But it was staying the course, and only his fears of future regret were heading into a death spiral.

"But the fact that you're going out on a limb like this to try it," Maya continued. "Spending your personal money and flying a plane yourself to pick it up... I just want you to know that I'm grateful for what you're doing. Maybe this *will* save Molly's life." She paused, her eyes locked intently on his. "And I know you did this for Jeremy's sake, too. That means a lot to me."

Cal wondered if Maya could see him visibly breathe a sigh of relief. Truth was, he had no qualms about putting a dent in his bank account to pay for the medicine. Many of his temporary gigs had included housing arrangements, which meant he'd been able to squirrel away most of his paychecks, and had a nice little nest egg to show for it. It was just money. And if it could buy Molly a second chance—something that he never had with Flaxxie, as much he'd wished had been the case so many times in the years since—then he'd happily spend every dime he had left.

He still had no way to know whether the drug would perform a late-stage miracle for Molly. But he *did* know that Maya was now on his side. Maybe she had been all along, but her protective instincts as a mother made her take pause at everything that had so quickly transpired. He couldn't blame her. If he were a father, he'd react the same way.

If I was a father...

Cal clenched his jaw as this thought reverberated in his head. He of all people should know that sometimes biological parents fell short—if they showed up at all—and those who stepped into the role could make all the difference in the life of a child.

And though he realized now might not be the best time to question his life choices, his brain took things one step further as he envisioned himself teaching Jeremy the ways of natural horsemanship with a fully healed Molly... Maya watching the three of them while leaning her arms over a fence, the biggest smile on her face...

Cal squeezed his eyes shut just long enough to bring himself back to the present. He turned to Maya, and this time, she was already facing him. As their eyes locked, her lips curved upward just enough to form the kind of smile that said *We're in this together*.

And suddenly, he no longer wondered why he'd been questioning his life choices.

CHAPTER TEN

CAL'S TRUCK HAD barely come to a stop before Maya threw open the passenger door and bolted out. She had already talked to her dad on the drive back from the airport, confirming that Molly was still hanging on. But she had suffered another seizure, and time was running out.

"Hurry!" she yelled back to Cal, despite knowing well that he didn't need to be prodded.

As she entered Molly's stall, her dad looked up, his expression grave. He glanced at Jeremy, still in the same spot against the stall wall with Cathy by his side, then back to Maya. She knew her dad didn't want to say anything too dire in front of Jeremy, but perhaps it was too late to pretend that this was no less than a life-or-death gamble.

Cathy's arm was wrapped tightly around Jeremy, and Maya managed an anxious smile in her direction to show her appreciation for looking after him in her absence.

"She's stable," Gus said in hushed tones as he ran a stethoscope over Molly's ribs, "or as stable as she can be, given her condition. I wasn't sure she was going to survive another seizure."

"Did you give more sedative?"

He nodded. "Forty-five minutes ago."

Maya bent down next to Molly and stroked her mane. She could almost feel the precarious dip in her life force, but *something* was still there. It was as if Molly knew they were trying to help her, and was clinging to life just long enough for them to return with the dorfamin.

Out of the corner of her eye, Maya could see that Cal had entered the stall and was setting up a portable IV infusion stand. "Four bags at a flow rate of eight hundred milligrams per hour," he said.

Gus looked up as he silently did the math in his head. "So roughly five hours."

"I'll stay with her tonight," Cal said as he came over and stooped down to hook the IV line up to her catheter.

"You don't think I'm actually going to leave—do you?" Maya asked incredulously.

Cal met her eyes and gave a quick nod, his smile unmistakable.

"Can I stay?" Jeremy called out, a question Maya knew she should've expected. But even so, she hadn't had a chance to fully think through her answer yet. It seemed unfair to send him home now, when he knew it was possible that Molly could pull through if the dorfamin worked. Still…just the sheer physical exhaustion of trying to stay awake all night was a lot for an eight-year-old boy.

"How about you stay in the house with me and get some sleep, and your mom and Cal can text us if anything happens?" Cathy asked, looking over at Maya with widened eyes as if to say, *I hope it's okay that I suggested this.*

"That's a great idea," Maya said, sharing a quick glance with Cal. His smile and nod indicated that he was on board with the plan as well.

"I don't want to miss anything," Jeremy said, his voice worried.

"I promise I'll let you guys know if you need to come out here."

"How about if I set the alarm for five hours from now, when the treatment ends?" Cathy suggested. "We'll come back out then, unless we hear from you before that."

"Perfect," Maya replied, walking over to kiss and hug Jeremy. "Get some sleep, honey. We'll take good care of Molly." Moments later, Cal was at her side, lowering himself onto one knee as he squeezed Jeremy's shoulder. "Molly knows you're rooting for her," he said quietly. "Get some rest like your mom said, and we'll see you in a bit."

Maya felt a stirring in her stomach as she watched Cal's genuine exchange with her son. Her emotions already heightened, she found it hard not to wish that their growing bond didn't have *temporary* stamped all over it.

Just like the deepening bond that you feel with Cal, too...

"How about if I bring out some blankets and a pot of coffee before I put on my pj's?" Cathy asked.

"That way, you can settle your tushes into something more comfy if you get tired."

Maya smiled, grateful for the chance to redirect her thoughts. "Thanks, Cathy. That would be great."

She waited for Cathy and Jeremy to exit the stall, then turned back to her dad. His eyes were focused downward on Molly, but even so, she could see the dark circles beneath them.

"Dad, why don't you go home and get some sleep. Sitting in a cold stall like this all night is only going to aggravate your arthritis."

Gus looked up at her, his shoulders heaving as he loudly sighed. "Did I mention that it sucks to get old?"

His reply drew laughter from both Maya and Cal, a brief respite from the unavoidable tension and heavy emotions that hung over all of them.

"I think I may have heard you say that once or twice before," Maya replied with a wry grin, reaching over to hug him and kiss him on the cheek.

Gus started to stand up, almost instantly staggering in midrise. Maya hopped to her feet and helped him straighten up, ignoring the tug on her ribs.

He thanked her, then looked over at Cal. "Well, I know Molly is in the best possible hands with the two of you. But you have to promise you'll call me if you need a third set of hands at any point." He held them up, and Maya discreetly winced at their gnarled knuckles and swollen finger joints. "They might have seen better days, but they're not fully out of commission yet."

"I promise."

Twenty minutes later, Maya scooched back from her kneeled position by Molly and turned to Cal, who was squatted down beside her. "If I don't stand up soon for a minute, I think my legs are going to start cramping."

He looked at her with a flash of concern. "I got this. Why don't you get up and walk around a bit. I'll join you in a few."

"Are you sure?"

He nodded to her, then again in the direction of the IV bag that hung from the infusion stand. "It looks like about a quarter of the bag has emptied, and no adverse reaction so far."

He stroked Molly's neck. Her eyes were half closed, her breathing slow and shallow. But she was still with them. Maya held her breath for a moment, as though exhaling too loudly might startle the mare. An entirely preposterous notion, she realized, but the stakes were so high, she'd do anything to stave off an anything-but-joyous outcome.

"Joe said the dorfamin would have an almost sedative-like effect while it's being administered, so as long as she stays subdued like this, we can hold off on any additional sedation."

Maya nodded. "Let's hope we can avoid that," she said, knowing well that adding sedation into *any* equation was bound to hike up the risk factor.

Spotting the blankets that Cathy had left earlier piled neatly up against the front stall wall, Maya headed over and eased her tired body down onto a floral-print comforter. A pot of coffee with two mugs rested on an overturned crate, but she resisted the urge to pour some for herself. Though physically spent, she was still mentally wired from the nonstop roller coaster of events that had defined the day. But once her adrenaline surge subsided, *then* it would be caffeine—and lots of it—to the rescue.

Pulling another blanket over her legs and waist to buffer against the nighttime chill, Maya leaned back against the wall as she watched Cal in action. Or inaction, given that he was immobile as he guarded over Molly while the treatment commenced. Either way, she could watch him for hours, touched by his unwavering dedication to his patients.

After some time had passed, she roused herself up and headed over to him.

"Hey," she said quietly. He'd been studying the dwindling level of dorfamin in the flowing IV bag, but quickly turned to her and smiled. "Hay is for horses."

She snickered, grateful for the tension-busting retort.

"So, what are you thinking?"

"We're about to start on the second bag, with two more to go." He looked down at Molly, and Maya did the same, making a mental note to recheck her vitals before the next IV bag was started. She was lying peacefully on her side...but that could be interpreted so many ways. And with an experimental drug, it was hard to know what was considered to be a "normal" presentation.

"This isn't based on anything other than my gut right now," Cal continued, "but I'm feeling optimistic."

Maya drew in a breath and held it several seconds before letting it out. "I trust your instincts. Your gut assessment is as good as gold in my book."

Cal looked both surprised and pleased by her comment.

Maya readied her stethoscope and knelt down by Molly's head, then looked back up at Cal. "Once you swap in the new bag, why don't you go sit down for a while and have some coffee. I can take over monitoring things."

"To be honest, I think as long as she's stable once we start the new bag, we can both sit back for a bit and let it work its magic."

A few minutes later, Cal examined the IV line with the new bag in place, nodding to confirm that everything was flowing smoothly.

"Shall we?" he asked with a half smile as he turned to Maya, gesturing toward the blankets.

Her heart skipped a beat as they walked over to the wall, and was downright pounding as he sat down on the floral comforter, then held up a corner of the top blanket so that she could slip underneath it and sidle up next to him.

Maya held her breath as she felt the heat of Cal's body seep into her own. He put his arm around her shoulders and pulled her in even closer. "You warm?"

She smiled and nodded. "Yes."

"Good."

Moments ticked by in silence. She'd been alone with Cal before. But not *alone* alone like they were now. Though a dim light from a ceiling fixture shone directly over Molly, the outskirts of the stall were darkened with shadows. Another few minutes of silence, then she discreetly turned to look at him, only to find that he was already staring at her.

"You know," he said, his voice a low whisper. "I've had some amazing, exhilarating experiences in my career as a vet, and there have been times when I would think to myself, 'I'll never forget this moment.' But right here, right now…waiting for a miracle to happen with you by my side…this moment tops them all."

Maya closed her eyes. If ever there was a moment that she too wanted to last forever…this was it. But could she tell him that? Seconds ticked by. Yes… yes, she could.

She opened her eyes and looked into his. "I feel the same way."

Even in the shadows, she could see a smile form on his face, but it was short-lived since he had other ideas for his lips—and hers.

His kiss quite literally took her breath away, but

she'd gladly trade oxygen for the chance to be this close to Cal, to feel his lips brush against hers, his strong body keeping her warmer than a thousand comforters ever could.

Maya awoke with a start, her face buried deep into something solid and warm. Only when she pulled her head away did she realize that the *something* was a fleece-covered nook between Cal's shoulder and chest. And then suddenly, everything came flooding back to her. Molly. An experimental treatment. *Oh—and Cal, cuddled underneath a blanket with me.*

Shaking herself fully awake, she looked up at him with widened eyes. "I can't believe I fell asleep."

He peered down at her with a half grin solidly in place. "That's okay. It's been a long night."

Maya jerked herself forward to get a better look at Molly, then blinked her eyes hard to make sure she wasn't imagining things. "Oh my god, she's sitting up!"

Cal's one-sided grin expanded into a full-on smile. "It happened about a half hour ago—just after you fell asleep, actually."

No longer lying flat out on her side, Molly had her four legs tucked beneath her belly, her head and shoulders fully raised off the ground.

Maya gasped. "Her head tilt is gone."

"I still can't believe it myself," Cal said quietly. Suddenly, his eyes widened. "Should we text Cathy to come out here with Jeremy?"

"Good idea," Maya said, pulling her phone out of her pocket. "They'll be out shortly," she said moments later. "I did tell Cathy they'll need to be very quiet when they enter the stall, so they don't startle her."

"Okay, good. From what I can see from here, there's less than a quarter of the last bag left to go. I think maybe we should sit tight, just to make sure the rest of it gets into her. Then we'll slowly approach her, remove the catheter and do an assessment."

Maya nodded in agreement. The good news was that Molly was awake and alert...but that also was the cautious news, given that she could decide to fully stand up at a moment's notice, potentially yanking out the IV catheter.

Several minutes later, the stall door creaked open. Cathy maneuvered Jeremy in front of her so that he could enter first. Maya put her finger to her lips and gently braced his shoulder with her other hand to halt him. He froze, then opened his eyes and mouth wide in shocked surprise as he spotted Molly's upright stance. The smile that emerged on his face, so pure and genuine and all-encompassing, grabbed Maya in the gut in the very best way. As Cal turned and witnessed the scene, he stood up beside them, his own smile bursting wide.

Suddenly, Molly nickered and pushed her front legs out from beneath her belly. Maya grabbed Cal's arm and gasped. He squeezed her hand and slowly moved up into a half-squatting position, ready to launch forward should Molly do the same.

In a flurry of shavings and snorts, Molly stood up, with Maya and Cal at her side before she had time to fully shake off the shavings that stuck to her hair.

"Let's keep her steady," Maya said, her eye on the nearly empty IV bag.

Cal gripped Molly's halter, talking to her in a low but still-affectionate voice. "Look at you, Molly. You are amazing…"

Drip…drip…drip…

Maya watched as the last drops of dorfamin emptied out of the bag and traveled down the IV line. A few more seconds, and then she removed the catheter from Molly's neck.

Too overcome with joy to utter a single word, Maya locked eyes with Cal, hoping he could read what she was thinking. But even her thoughts were tongue-tied.

We did it! No—you did it! Molly did it! Make that—we all did it!

Cal grinned, an expression she'd seen on his face many times before, but never with such intensity.

Maya turned back to Jeremy. Cathy's arm was stretched across his chest, as though ready to hold him back, should he try to run over to Molly too soon.

"You guys can come over. Just walk slowly," Maya said softly.

As Jeremy nimbly approached, Cathy waited

back, as though giving him the opportunity to have a moment alone with Molly.

He reached up and petted her nose, then turned to Maya and threw his arms around her waist. Before she could fully react, he turned to Cal and did the same, but in this instance, there was no letting go.

"Thank you, Cal! You saved Molly..." Tears streamed down his face as he looked up at Cal. "You saved her!"

Maya rubbed her eyes with the sleeve of her jacket. In veterinary medicine, as in the human kind, one had to put personal emotions on hold. At least, that had been the adage drummed into her from her earliest days in veterinary college. *You won't be able to survive the sheer number of disappointments otherwise*, she'd been told time and again.

But that wasn't going to happen today. Her emotions were too raw...and yes, too personal.

As Cal looked over at her, still locked in an embrace with Jeremy, she caught her breath at the expression on his face. He wasn't just hugging Jeremy back in a perfunctory manner. No—there was real emotion there, and it seemed to go beyond feeling glad that his horse-saving actions had made someone ecstatically happy.

He almost looked...fatherly.

Maya briefly closed her eyes, warning herself not to go there. And where exactly was *there*? It was any colorful scenario she was conjuring up in her mind that glossed over the black-and-white truth:

Cal was strictly a colleague, and a temporary one at that. Which meant any perceived affection toward her or her son—regardless of how genuine—was equally transitory, and it would be a grave mistake to ever think otherwise.

Except...the "black-and-white truth" had morphed into something grayer. Her deepening connection with Cal was making it nearly impossible to continue seeing him as a temporary colleague only. Or, for that matter, a temporary colleague with whom she shared a real but going-nowhere attraction. *We're past that point.* The question was...did he feel the same?

CHAPTER ELEVEN

Maya pulled into the parking lot of the practice barn and clinic, ready to start another day with a spring in her step. Nearly a week had passed since Molly's nothing-short-of-miraculous turnaround, and the happy ending seemed to have buoyed the spirits of everyone involved in her recovery.

Not that she didn't have reason to still hold on to a snippet of caution. Just due to their sheer strength and size, horses were often thought to be hearty and resilient in the face of illness, but that was far from the truth. Even the slightest dietary changes could set off a deadly case of colic, and up until fairly recently, a leg break—so treatable in other animals—almost inevitably led to euthanasia.

But spotting Cal's truck as she hopped out of her own, Maya was back in Happyville again. Entering the barn, she ran through the day's tasks in her head. A hoof laminitis case at 9:00 a.m. A blood draw for a metabolic blood panel at 10:30 a.m….a hindgut ulcer consult at noon…

It was quiet as she walked down the aisle while ruminating on her to-do list—emphasis on *was*. Suddenly, the washroom door flew open, and in a flash of brawny flesh, a shirtless Cal came charging out. He skidded to a halt as he came chest-to-face with Maya.

"Oh," he said, wide-eyed.

"Oh," she replied, wider-eyed.

All together now: "*Oh!*"

He looked down at where his shirt should be, saying, "I was syringing Fern with dewormer paste, and she spit it back out on me."

"Well, at least you don't have to worry about carrying around a tapeworm."

Maya squinted her eyes shut. *Did I actually say that?* There was something about seeing Cal with no shirt and...*gulp*...all muscle that put her brain, and other body parts, in a tizzy.

Cal laughed heartily. "Not my first thought when she spit on me, I'll say that. But can't argue with the logic."

As he took a step toward her, she tripped a step back. But it was a *teensy-weensy* step, because apparently even her feet knew a good thing when they saw one.

"Someone's going to see us," Maya said breathlessly as he pulled her close and nuzzled her neck.

"Only Fern," he whispered as the feisty thoroughbred stuck her head over the stall gate.

A half dozen other horses followed suit, but Maya paid little heed. It was the first time she was ever glad that horses couldn't talk.

"We can't cross that line again—remember?" she

said almost dreamily, doing very little to actually halt said crossing.

"You mean this line?" he asked softly as he play-bit her bottom lip.

Uh huh...

He pulled the bottom of her shirt out of her jeans, and she did little to stop him. Correction—she did *nothing* to upend the pleasurable sensations that were welling up inside her. His hands caressed her back, sending shivers down the length of her body. As they moved to the front, she caught her breath, startled by the sound of her own gasp.

Or was something else tugging at her ears?

She pulled back slightly. "Wait—is that a car I hear?"

Cal froze as well, turning an ear toward the open barn entrance. "Is a client scheduled to come by?"

"No. Hold on a sec." She scurried over just in time to see her dad exiting his SUV and looking toward the barn. "Oh no—it's my dad!"

Maya took a deep breath, reminding herself that she was not a little girl anymore, and if she wanted to canoodle with her hunky colleague in the barn aisle...*then that's my prerogative!*

Still, a bare-chested Cal would be hard to explain.

"Hurry—put your shirt on!" she whisper-shouted.

"I can't! It's soaking in the sink."

Maya grabbed her head with both hands to think, accidentally clunking herself with her cast in the process. "All right. Look—all we have to do is tell the truth."

Cal balked. "That we were making out?"

"No! That you had to take your shirt off because of Fern." She grabbed his arm and pulled him forward. "Let's go. We need to cut this off at the quick!"

Her directive, both serious and intentionally humorous at the same time, prompted a nervous chuckle from Cal.

Nearly stumbling out together into the morning sun, Maya greeted her dad with a chirpy "Hi!" that sounded one note higher than Alvin the Chipmunk.

Cal's not-so-discreet nudge at her side alerted her to the fact that her shirt was askew, one half tucked into her jeans and the other half flailing about. Clearing her throat, she pulled the tucked half out, hoping it would be less obvious than pushing everything back in. Judging by the quizzical expression on her dad's face, it wasn't.

He looked at Maya, then at Cal, then at Maya, then at Cal.

That's quite the head swivel, Maya thought as she tried to pull back on a teeth-baring grimace.

"*Callll?*" her dad began, eyes narrowed while drawing out the name as though it had twelve letters instead of three.

Cal cleared his throat. "Yes, Mr. Evans?"

"I've told you before to call me Gus—remember?"

"Yes, Mr. Gus—" Cal immediately shook his head. "—I mean, yes, Gus?"

"Is there a reason why you're not wearing a shirt in fifty-degree weather?"

"Fern spit dewormer paste on him," Maya hurriedly interjected.

"What she said," Cal added, pointing to Maya in case it wasn't clear who *she* was.

Gus studied him further, mouth twisted to the side and eyes in a tight squint. "Huh. Well, I do have some clean shirts in the office if you want to borrow one." He held his lanky arms out in front of himself and inspected them closely, then homed in on Cal's brawny physique. "Although, you might have to take a scalpel to the sleeves if your arms are going to fit through them."

Maya bowed her head in a muffled snicker.

She turned to Cal, whose reddened cheeks told her he'd be sweating under his shirt if he was actually wearing one. Instead, he nervously shifted his weight from one foot to the other. "Thanks. But I have a change of clothes in my truck. Kind of a necessity with this job."

Gus slowly eased into a smile, signaling to Maya that she could breathe again. "It is, isn't it."

Suddenly, the door to the office across the way opened and Jeremy strode out, a red lollipop from a bowl on Maria's desk in hand.

"Jeremy!" Maya exclaimed. "What are you doing here? Why aren't you at school?"

"I was about to get to that," Gus said. "There was

a water pipe break at the school, and the students were sent home."

She turned to her son. "Why didn't you ask the school to call me?"

"I asked them to call Grandpa to come get me because I knew you were working."

Maya's tense shoulders eased up a bit. "Oh, okay, that makes sense."

"I know Carla could look after him today," Gus began, "but I figured he'd be bored at home all day, so he's going to tag along with me on some errands."

"Thanks, Dad." She turned back to Jeremy. "Although, my day is mostly standard appointments, so you can come with me if you'd rather do that."

He looked over at Cal. "Can I go with you, instead?"

Maya started to open her mouth, but wasn't sure what should come out. She hadn't seen this question coming...but perhaps she should have.

"That's fine with me," Cal said, turning to Maya with slight apprehension in his eyes. "But only if it's okay with your mom."

In a way, she couldn't blame her son for wanting to spend the day with Cal. Heck—she'd do the same, if it weren't for the fact that they were splitting up appointments today.

She could imagine Jeremy's thought process on the matter. *Do I spend the day with my*—yawn!—*predictable mom, or with Cal, the Indiana Jones of the horse world?*

"Are you sure?" she asked Cal, wondering if he could sense how difficult it was for her to navigate Jeremy's growing attachment to him. "I know you have a couple of surgical procedures scheduled."

"I'm excising a skin growth and stitching up a gash. Nothing too complicated." Cal turned to Jeremy with a wink and a grin. "And we can probably squeeze in a visit to see Molly. How does that sound?"

Jeremy let out a loud gasp. "Awesome!"

Maya felt her lips curve into a smile. Few things could bring her as much joy as seeing her son's unfiltered happiness. But her smile wavered as another truth set in. The stronger that Jeremy's bond with Cal grew, the harder it was going to be for him when Cal inevitably moved on.

And harder for you, too.

Maya pushed the obviousness from her thoughts. Maybe she would need to reevaluate how much one-on-one time Jeremy should have with Cal, but right now, she was not going to spoil his excitement.

Loading her truck for the day after Cal had set off for his own set of appointments with Jeremy, Maya turned to pick up a portable X-ray machine and nearly jumped to find her dad quietly standing just inches away. "You scared me!"

"Sorry."

She cocked her head to the side, reading the concern on his face almost too easily. "Is there something you want to say?" she asked, figuring it was best to just get things out in the open.

"Not really," he replied unconvincingly.

She silently coaxed him with raised eyebrows.

"Maya, you're a grown woman, and what goes on in your personal life is your own business. The only thing that matters to me is that you're happy. And Jeremy, too, of course. The two of you mean the world to me."

Maya heard his "not my business" words, but his troubled eyes told another story.

"But…" she prodded.

He opened his mouth as if to speak, then stopped and shook his head. "Nothing."

"No—tell me, Dad."

"I had a call yesterday from a vet clinic in England, of all places. They were checking references for Cal. Seems like he's already started searching for his next job."

The revelation pulled all the oxygen out of Maya's lungs, and it took several moments to recover her breath. She steadied herself with the reminder that nothing her dad had just said should have come as a surprise. Cal wasn't doing something devious behind her back. He was merely making plans to ensure that he stayed employed *somewhere*—as well he should.

"Well, that's understandable—right?" she quickly countered. "The contract that you had him sign was for two months. I'm sure he's just trying to line something up now, so he won't have a long gap of unemployment when his time here is done."

"You're right. Which is why I wasn't going to say anything. But—and maybe I'm just imagining things—it seems like you and Cal have grown closer recently, and it's obvious that Jeremy thinks the world of him, too." He paused, a "should I say more?" look on his face. "I just don't want to see you guys get hurt like you did when Max left."

"This is different," Maya said, though she knew well that her dad had a valid point. "I was in a long-term relationship with Max."

Gus pursed his lips together and nodded, then reached over and gently squeezed Maya's shoulder. "You're right. I'm just being a silly, overprotective dad who needs to mind his own business. In fact, I can hear your mom looking down on us right now and saying, 'Goddamn it, Gus, leave poor Maya alone. Let her live her life.'"

Maya snickered, though she knew her mom *would* be saying those exacts words if she were here. But at the same time…she'd probably also find an unobtrusive way to share her concerns as well.

"I appreciate you looking out for me, Dad, I really do. But I'll be okay, and so will Jeremy. I'll make sure of that."

He smiled. "I know you will."

As Maya watched his SUV head down the driveway and onto the main road a short time later, she wondered why his words of reassurance only made her feel worse.

Was she making sure that she and Jeremy would be okay? Her actions, both in the barn earlier with Cal, and then allowing Jeremy to tag along with him for the day, seemed to suggest otherwise. And though she had outwardly tried to casually shrug off her dad's revelation about Cal's job inquiry, inwardly she was still reeling.

Maybe she *was* getting too caught up in a fantasy notion of what she and Jeremy meant to Cal. And the one thing about fantasies? They eventually all came to an end.

Unless…was it possible he had applied for the job early on, before their growing closeness?

Maya took a deep breath, then continued loading her truck. She couldn't definitively answer that question—at least not yet.

Cal pulled his truck into the long driveway leading to Maya's house, coming to a stop in front of the large, wraparound porch. He was surprised to see her truck parked in front as well, given that it was 4:45 p.m., and she had mentioned her last appointment was at 5:00 p.m.

"Thanks, Cal," Jeremy said, opening the passenger door. "I can't wait to tell my mom that we saw Molly."

Cal smiled, a feeling of *all is right in the world* coursing through his veins.

Hokey, much? he wanted to ask himself. Except that the feeling was too genuine...and too full of goodness...for him to want to tear it down.

"I thought you'd still be on rounds," he said to Maya as she came out to greet them from the top of the porch steps. She dodged to the side as Jeremy rushed past. "Rusty inside?" he asked, already through the front door before she fully had a chance to answer.

"Slow down!" she exclaimed affectionately before turning back to Cal. "My last appointment had to reschedule. Ten sheath cleanings at Mountain Acres Farm. Can't say I'm disappointed."

Cal was surprised that Maya put that image into his head of her slathering cream over ten horse penises, but perhaps he was letting his powers of visualization get the best of him. Still, he shuddered slightly before scanning her property. With trees at the height of autumn colors, rolling fields still pre-frost green and a backdrop of mist-covered mountains, it was hard not to be moved by nature at its most glorious.

"It's beautiful out here," he observed. "I didn't see much when I picked you up for the fundraiser because it was dark. But you have a lot more land than I realized."

"Ten acres," Maya confirmed as she stepped down off the porch.

Cal stretched his neck to get a better look at a

large structure off in the distance. "Is that a barn back there?"

Maya nodded. "Twenty stalls, believe it or not. Plus three fenced pastures."

"And no horses of your own?"

"Kind of doesn't add up—right?" Maya acknowledged, scrunching her lips together for emphasis. "Horse vet with a barn and pastures…and no horses."

"Well, not like you have a ton of free time to care for them if you did, I suppose."

"Free time? What's that?" Maya flashed a wry grin, but it was quickly followed by a sigh of resignation. "Truth is, I'd always planned to get horses when I moved here. But this place was a bit of a fixer-upper—especially the barn and fencing. George and I…" She paused momentarily, as though wondering whether it was appropriate to bring her late husband into the conversation. "We talked about starting a sanctuary for unwanted horses. We knew how Cathy had to turn some away because she had no room. But…we weren't even here half a year before he died, so all those plans came to a halt." She paused again, pulling her lips in tight before forcing the hint of a smile. "Anyway, someday I'll get to the repairs."

"What kind of repairs are we talking about?" Cal asked, ready to throw a workbag full of tools over his shoulder. Not that he actually had one—yet.

"Well, the barn has a leaky roof, and the electricity's not working. Some of the stall gates need to be replaced, too."

"Are there at least a couple working stalls?"

"There are, but there are some major breaks in the fencing that would need to be repaired before I could house any horses here. To be honest, with enough time and money, it's all doable stuff that could be fixed in a probably a week or two. I had planned to hire someone, but then Max came into my life and insisted he'd help me get everything up to speed..." She paused, her train of thought hitting a roadblock. "Well, let's just say that never happened. And between his leaving the practice, and my dad having to cut back his hours, I've had to put this on the back burner." There was a faraway look in her eyes as she viewed the bucolic surroundings. "But someday," she quietly added.

The front door opened and Jeremy emerged with a full backpack hanging off one shoulder.

"Where do you think you're going?" Maya asked.

"Mark's for dinner. I told you yesterday—it's his birthday."

As if on cue, a car slowly rambled up the driveway. Maya looked at Cal, her brow furrowed, then turned to wave to Mark's parents as the vehicle came to a stop in front of her.

"Hold on!" she exclaimed, halting Jeremy midstride to the car. "What time are you coming home?"

"I'm staying over—I told you that, too."

Maya shook her head in bewilderment. "There's

been so much going on, I forgot all about it. Well, have fun—and be careful!"

Cal waited for the car to disappear from view, then turned back to Maya. Was he going to take advantage of this sudden development? *Heck, yeah!*

"Well, looks like it's just the two of us. How does dinner sound?"

"It sounds good," Maya replied a little too quickly. "I'm reheating lasagna from the other night. What about you?"

"I'm cooking some burgers on the grill on my deck. Care to join me?"

"I can't," Maya replied a little too quickly. "I'm a vegetarian—not sure if I ever mentioned that to you. So, veggie burgers only."

Oh, you aren't going to push me off that easily...
"Not a problem. We'll pick some up on the way."

If ever there was a make-or-break moment, this had to be it, Maya thought. Her decision now could reverberate for a long time to come…unless, of course, Cal simply just wanted to cook her a veggie burger. Although judging by the hungry look in his eyes, there's was potentially more on the menu than dinner.

Still…as long as she made a pledge with herself to simply enjoy the present moment and rein in her emotions…then there was no harm in throwing a little caution to the wind. *Right?*

"Okay," she said, pushing her doubts back and a smile forth.

Twenty minutes later, they entered Cal's cabin, grocery bags in hand. "It's chilly in here," Cal said. "I'll start a fire."

Crackling orange flames added a warm glow to the already-cozy living room as he headed back over to the adjoining kitchen.

Maya pulled out a stool to sit at the counter, but paused as Cal looked at her quizzically and said, "Something's different..."

She grinned and held up her left arm. "I was wondering how long it would take you to notice."

His eyes widened. "You got your cast off!"

"This afternoon—finally!"

"How does your arm feel?"

"A little weird, to be honest. I'm used to having the weight of the cast, but I'm sure that will quickly pass."

As Cal closed the space between them and gently touched her arm, she held her breath. His blue-green eyes locked on to hers, and all her inner protests, the can't do this, shouldn't do this, will live to regret it proclamations, slowly melted away.

"Does this make it feel better?" he asked, lifting her arm, his eyes still locked on to hers, and then kissing the inside of her wrist.

Maya silently gasped and closed her eyes, her knees nearly buckling as desire flooded through her. As Cal's lips moved to her neck and then her lips, she grabbed on to his shoulders to steady herself, then clasped his neck as he suddenly picked her up and quite literally swept her off her feet.

Time stood still as he carried her into the bedroom. A large fur blanket was draped over the queen-size bed, and as he laid her down on top of it, he softly added, "Don't worry, it's faux fur. I checked."

Damn, this man really knows me...

And it wasn't just knowing how her mind worked. With every sensuous kiss, every scintillating touch, he blissfully brought her to places that she never could have imagined. It was as if they'd been lovers forever.

And yet...as they basked in the afterglow of their lovemaking, Maya couldn't help but think how *forever* was the one thing she'd never truly have with Cal.

"Are you sorry we crossed the line?" he asked with a slightly mischievous grin, kissing her on the forehead as he stroked her arm.

Maya smiled and gently shook her head. But the answer in her thoughts?

In this moment, no, but tomorrow, which will be one day closer to you leaving for good...maybe.

CHAPTER TWELVE

"THERE'S NO EASY way to say this...but I have cancer."

Sitting across from Cathy, Cal felt his insides plunge. As Maya gasped and grabbed his knee, he placed his hand over hers and held it tight. Earlier that day, Cathy had called to ask that they stop by together, and though she cryptically left out a reason for her request, never in a million years did Cal expect such a devastating announcement.

"Cathy—" Maya began, seemingly too shocked to say anything more.

"I know. You thought I was an invincible Wonder Woman, right? I thought so, too—minus the big boobs and curves."

Though Cathy smiled wryly at her attempt to diffuse the gravity of her announcement with humor, Maya's face remained stricken. She glanced at Cal, whose face was equally grave.

"Truth is, I haven't been feeling well for a while. Couldn't really put my finger on it, just an overall sense of fatigue, sometimes breathlessness. But given that I'm pushing seventy, I kept writing it off as old... I mean, as less-than-young age. My doctor ran some tests, and turns out I have Hodgkin's lymphoma. The good news is we caught it fairly early. But I'm still looking at several rounds of chemotherapy, possibly followed by radiation treatment.

"And if I *were* younger, I'd figure I'll beat this and then come back stronger than ever. I'm still going to do everything I can to kick this cancer to the curb, but I can't kid myself. It's been getting harder to do all the physical work of taking care of the horses, and even if I hired help—which I really can't afford—the upkeep of a place this size is more than I'm going to be able to handle. My sister Karen has offered to let me stay with her while I'm going through the treatments, and then once I'm on the other side of that, I can look for my own place, something smaller and more manageable."

"Cathy, I'm so sorry," Maya said, her voice quivering.

Cathy leaned over and grabbed both of Maya's hands. "No crying now. You hear me? I'm going to get through this. And what's going to help me do that is knowing that my horses are going to good homes."

Maya glanced at Cal, and he knew what she was thinking. *Where exactly are these homes?* The reason that rescues like Happy Hooves existed in the first place was because it was so hard to find caring and qualified people willing to take on the time and expense of caring for a horse.

"Have you thought of selling the rescue to someone who'd take it over?" Maya asked. "And by that, I mean someone who'd continue your mission of rescuing horses, or at least caring for the ones you have now."

"Believe me, I thought about that, and I put out some feelers to some local real estate agents. But it's a tough sell. I mean, let's face it—running a rescue is a lot of work, and the money to keep it going is always an issue. If it weren't for the generosity of you and your dad over the years with all the pro-bono vet care, Happy Hooves would probably have fallen under a long time ago."

Maya hung her head downward, and Cal could almost feel the despair emanating off her. As he squeezed her hand, she turned to him with a sadness in her eyes that felt like a knife in his own heart.

"Are you okay?" he asked on the drive back to her house, his question piercing a long stretch of silence.

"Not really. Cathy has always been such a strong person and a tremendous advocate for horses that I never thought this day would come. And in case you're wondering, don't think my mind didn't jump to the barn and fields on my property. But running a rescue is a lot of work, and I don't think I can realistically take that on by myself on top of my job and Jeremy…not to mention that part of my property would need a major upgrade first."

"I wasn't wondering that," Cal said quietly. "I already know how much you're carrying on your shoulders." He paused, glancing at her sideways. "Your *tiny* shoulders, I should add."

"They're still big enough to have helped pull Buttercup up off the ground."

Cal could see the effort behind her slight smile. "True that."

Maya's smile faded as she looked out the passenger window. "You know, when I was a little girl, tagging along with my dad on client visits… I remember going to Happy Hooves and thinking that someday, I'd have my own horse rescue."

"Maybe you will, when the time is right."

She glossed over his suggestion. "I guess all we can do right now is get the word out to clients about the horses being up for adoption."

He reached over and brushed away a loose lock of hair that obscured the side view of her face. She turned to him abruptly, eyes momentarily surprised, then clasped his hand and brought it up to her lips.

The soft kiss on his knuckles still hit him hard… because it was so much more than a kiss. It was a confirmation that she knew she could lean on him. He'd do anything to be there for her, to be the rock that had long been missing in her life.

And what happens to that rock when you up and leave in a month?

Cal ignored his own question.

The sun was just starting to set when they arrived back at Maya's place. He pulled the truck up in front of the house, leaving the engine idling as he turned to her.

"Thanks for picking me up," she said, her troubled eyes saying more than her words.

"Of course."

Another span of silence. "Well, I'll see you in the morning."

Maya hopped off the passenger seat before Cal could reply, but instead of closing the truck door behind her, she froze with her back facing him.

Seconds ticked by, and he wondered whether to ask if she was okay. Just as his mouth started forming the words, she swiftly turned around.

"Do you want to come in for dinner? I'm just heating up a casserole that Carla prepared earlier, but she's a much better cook than me, and it's way more food than Jeremy and I can finish alone."

Cal greeted the invitation with a slightly agape mouth and widened eyes. On the one hand, it was simply an on-the-spot dinner invitation. But on the other, it had to have come with a heaping serving of trust on Maya's behalf. He knew how closely she guarded her homelife with Jeremy.

"I'd love to," he replied.

Cal followed Maya into the living room, surprising Jeremy as he did. He'd been tussling on the carpeted floor with a large golden retriever, who froze and barked at Cal's presence.

"It's okay, Rusty," Maya said. Her reassurance was all the dog needed to snap out of attention and resume playing with Jeremy.

"Cal's joining us for dinner tonight," Maya said.

Jeremy greeted the news with a huge smile and a thumbs-up.

Cal looked around the living room and adjoining kitchen, impressed with what he saw. He was no Martha Stewart, but if he had to put a label on the decor, he guessed it would be "modern country."

"I don't have any beer," Maya called over as she pulled two wineglasses out of a cabinet. "But would you like a glass of wine?"

"Sure." He felt something rub up against his leg, then leaned over to pet an orange tiger cat.

"Wow," Maya said as she looked over. "Willow almost never comes out when company is here. She must know you're an animal lover."

Cal grinned. "Win over the cats, and everything else is a piece of cake."

Maya laughed. "There's definitely some truth to that." She headed over and handed him a glass of merlot. "It won't take long to heat up the casserole."

"I'm in no rush," he said, which was the understatement of the year. They hadn't even sat down to eat yet, but just being in her home, with Jeremy playing with his dog, Maya sipping wine while readying dinner, a cat—now two—circling him affectionately... If was as if the term *domestic bliss* had suddenly sprung to life and pulled him into the center of it.

It was the quintessential family home life he didn't know he needed. Or...did he in fact already know? Not having something and not wanting it were two different things. He'd had a taste of this sense of belonging with Thomas and Mabel at the ranch, albeit with a bitter ending that had soured him on ever pursuing a lasting attachment again.

Yet, slowly but surely, this previously wrought iron resolve was beginning to crumble. He could feel it in every fiber of his being, in every pang of *I don't want this to end* that grabbed at him each time he thought about leaving Maya.

But it *had* to be this way...or did it? Just because running away had always worked for him in the past, did that mean there was no other option now? What if he wanted more? A life with Maya and Jeremy? The *what-ifs* continued to circle his mind with no answer in sight, perhaps because he'd never asked them before.

It was dark as Cal and Maya retreated to the porch to finish their glasses of wine.

"I can't remember the last time I had a delicious, home-cooked meal like that," Cal said as he seated himself on a cushioned wicker bench.

Maya sat down beside him. "You mean a home-heated-up meal," she replied with a wry smile. "But it *was* cooked from scratch earlier in the day, courtesy of Carla."

He chuckled, his easy laughter tapering off as a deeper revelation crept into his thoughts. Sitting at the dinner table earlier with Maya and Jeremy... talking and laughing and just being themselves...he couldn't think of a better way to end the day. No—

that wasn't quite right. He couldn't think of a better way to end *every* day.

The distinction caught Cal hard in the gut, and he turned to Maya with what he realized too late had to be a deer-in-the-headlights look on his face.

"What's wrong?" she asked, forehead creased and eyebrows raised.

"Nothing." He silently caught his breath in an effort to hide his angst, adding in a forced smile to boot. "Nothing at all."

Which, of course, wasn't exactly true. Because in about a month from now, he'd be packing up his bags on the way to his next gig. That was the contract he'd signed—happily and willingly—at the start of his temporary employment with Northern Vermont Equine Associates. The sort of contract he insisted on, no matter where the wind had taken him.

Which was all fine and dandy, except for the fact that the wind had last deposited him *here*…right smack in the midst of a woman he could truly fall for.

Could truly fall for? As in it hadn't happened yet? Who in the world was he kidding? He wouldn't have been questioning his gig-hopping ways just a short time ago if Maya was like all the other colleagues—female or otherwise—whom he'd easily moved on from in the past with little more than the flick of a departing handwave.

Yes, this was all new to him. Yes, it was scary. But perhaps he could take a few baby steps before attempting to jump feetfirst into a life of happiness that had always seemed out of his reach, but was closer now than ever before.

He cleared his throat, readying for that first tiny step. "We'll have to do this again. How about if I cook dinner for you and Jeremy at my place tomorrow night? You can bring Rusty and the cats. We'll make it a family affair."

He expected Maya to laugh at his comment, but instead, she stared at the ground, looking one step short of stricken.

"Did I say something wrong?" he gingerly asked.

It took her a moment to reply. "Cal—I know I'm the one who asked you to stay for dinner, but I'm not sure that I thought things through enough. After learning about Cathy's situation…it felt good having you by my side, like I wasn't facing such horrible news alone. I guess I wanted to continue that feeling once we got back here. But relying on you like this…that's just going to make it harder when you leave."

"Maya…" He wanted to say more, but knew he'd only be digging a deeper hole for himself. It wasn't as though he could counteract any points that she had just made. And there were more points to come.

"You have to understand—I'm not like you. The whole 'I'll land wherever the wind takes me' thing—that's just not me."

Cal's eyes widened. He didn't remember using

that phrase in front of her before. But maybe it was written on his persona.

"I don't get attached to many people," she continued. "It's just the way I am—maybe it's in part a protection thing. But when I do…it's not…"

"It's not what?" he asked, nudging her after a lapse of silence ensued.

"It's not a temporary feeling that I can just shrug off when the person is no longer in my life." She paused, searching his eyes. "Do you understand what I mean?"

He nodded, unable to say more.

"And the fact that you're able to leave one job—or one continent, for that matter—at a moment's notice while heading to another, tells me you're not like this."

"Maya—"

"Please, let me finish. I can't imagine you haven't met women along the way who you've become involved with."

Cal clenched his jaw. There was involved, and then there was *involved*. A distinction that was clear in his mind, but it would only make matters worse if he tried to explain this to Maya.

"And it's not just about me. Jeremy has gotten close to you, too. And yes, he's older now than when he was with the whole Max fiasco—and I'm not trying to imply that we're in any sort of relationship like I was with Max, because we're not."

Cal wondered if Maya knew how skillful she was

with a dagger. She wasn't *intentionally* skewering him, of course. But her words pierced him sharply just the same.

"But it will still be very hard on Jeremy when you leave. And even more so if he thinks there's a chance that you'll stay. I told him when you were hired that it was just for a couple of months. But I don't think he's looking at it that way right now." She paused. "You know how kids are—they live in the present."

Cal couldn't recall ever being at a total loss for words as he was now. But what could he possibly say? It wasn't a stretch to put himself in Maya's shoes and realize that as a mother, and as a woman who'd already experienced her share of romantic heartbreak, everything she'd said made sense. She was protecting herself and her son.

Think about that. You want to protect her...but she needs protection from you.

"Maya, it's not like I have one foot out the door—"

"Really?" she asked pointedly. "Because my dad mentioned he was recently contacted as a reference for a job in England."

Cal froze. *She knows.* He had applied for a four-month gig in the Cotswolds to cover an upcoming maternity leave only days after arriving in Vermont. With this new role scheduled to start a couple weeks after his current contract ended, it had seemed like perfect timing. Emphasis on *seemed*. But that was before his growing feelings for Maya. When he'd received an email the night before confirming that he was moving forward in the hiring process, the normally happy news had actually filled him with a sense of dread.

But even if he tried to explain this to Maya, she wouldn't believe him. Besides, what would he say? *Yeah, I hate to have to leave, but I'm going to do it anyway.* Because that was always the bottom line with him, wasn't it?

Except…the line was beginning to shift. And yet, as he looked into Maya's eyes, he felt too paralyzed to do anything about it. He knew what he was feeling…for Maya, for the life they could have together…but perhaps it was too big of a leap. He thought he could start with baby steps, but with Maya laying it all out on the line like this, he couldn't even stick out a toe. Whether it was due to fear of failure, or just plain fear, it almost didn't matter at this point.

As if sensing his inner turmoil, Maya took a deep breath, her voice now softened. "I didn't mean to end this night on such a sour note—especially after such a difficult day. I just wanted us to be clear on a few things for the remainder of your time here."

He nodded. "I appreciate your honesty."

Which he did. The question was…could he be honest with himself?

CHAPTER THIRTEEN

MAYA WATCHED AS her dad drove up the clinic driveway with Jeremy in tow. Two days had passed since she and Cal had received Cathy's devastating news, and between this and Cal's imminent departure, she was having a hard time finding reasons to smile.

But seeing Jeremy's excitement as he bounded out of the SUV temporarily put her angst on hold. Her dad had promised to take him to see Molly after school, and it was clear that the visit had been a positive one.

"How's she doing?" Maya asked, smiling for the first time all day.

"I got to pet her!" Jeremy exclaimed, which prompted her smile to widen even more.

"That's great, honey."

"I'm going to get a lollipop," he said.

"Just one—cavities, remember?"

He rolled his eyes, then nodded before heading to the office.

Maya turned to her dad as he came up beside her. "Don't worry. Cathy didn't say anything about the cancer or closing the rescue in front of Jeremy."

She breathed a sigh of relief. "I know we can't keep the truth from him forever, but I want it to be done the right way. It's a lot for someone his age to take in, and I want to sit down with him and explain everything."

Her dad nodded. "I agree."

"I know the first thing he's going to ask is what will happen to Molly."

"Did you talk to Cathy yet about adopting her?"

"Not yet," Maya said with a sigh. "She started chemo yesterday and I don't want to throw too much at her right now. I'm also not going to say anything to Jeremy about the adoption until I've ironed out all the details. If we take in Molly, we should adopt a second horse as a companion. There's no way I can completely overhaul the barn and fencing right now, so I need to figure out the minimum that needs to be done to get things up to speed. For two horses, it shouldn't be too bad."

"I'm sure Cal would be willing to help."

Maya didn't disagree with her dad's assessment, but the bigger question was whether having Cal around her home, helping out more like a partner than a fellow vet, would be too misleading for Jeremy. *Or for me*.

But before she could share such concerns with her dad, she turned to the sound of Cal's truck heading up the driveway.

As he slid out of the driver's seat moments later, Australian cowboy hat in place, dark blond hair scraping his shoulders and sturdy cowboy boots firmly on the ground, Maya's heart fluttered.

Don't do that, she reprimanded it. And still, it fluttered again.

Jeremy had just exited the office with a lollipop in hand, and spotting Cal, immediately ran over to him. "Hey, Cal—guess who I saw today?"

"Let's see…was it someone with two legs or four?"

"Four!" Jeremy exclaimed, game to play along.

"Tail or no tail?"

"Tail!"

"Black, white, red or brown?"

"Brown—but really light brown."

Cal's grin widened. "I'm going to take a wild guess here and say Molly."

Jeremy lifted his small hand in a high five, which Cal quickly but gently slapped.

Maya exchanged a curious glance with her dad. "Since when does Jeremy high-five people?"

"Apparently since he's met Cal," her dad replied with a light chuckle.

"Grandpa said that come spring, Molly should be strong enough to start building up her muscles again. I want to learn how to lunge her and stuff. Do you think you'll be able to show me?"

Cal had been straightening out supplies in the back of his truck, but slowed to a halt as he fielded Jeremy's question. He briefly turned to Maya, then looked away as if he knew she was holding her breath for his answer. Which, in fact, she was.

"I think it might be a little too soon to start her

on a lunge line," Cal said, swinging the truck doors shut and turning to give Jeremy his full attention.

"I don't mean now. But can you show me in the spring?"

"I, um…" Cal's stammered nonreply was like a jackhammer to Maya's heart.

This was the scenario she'd been dreading, and now it was playing out in real time before her.

"Jeremy, honey," Maya said as she slowly approached, "Cal's probably not going to be here in the spring."

Of course, she knew that *probably* was actually *definitely*, but she couldn't quite bring herself to unleash the harsh reality full force upon her son.

The shock on Jeremy's face, first aimed at her until he whipped his head in Cal's direction, knocked the wind out of her.

"Where are you going?" he asked, his voice rising.

"I'm not sure yet. Probably England." Cal paused, momentarily locking eyes with Maya before turning back to Jeremy. "The job here was just for a couple of months, to help your mom while she was healing from the horse kick."

Jeremy turned to Maya, eyes darting to her dad and then back to her. "But don't you still need another vet now that Grandpa's retiring?"

Maya flinched as she felt her father's hand on her shoulder from behind, her head quite literally buzzing as high-pressured blood whooshed through her ears.

"Jeremy, Cal's a traveling vet." She had no idea if he ever ascribed to this label himself—but she also didn't care. Right now, her only priority was to soften the blow of Cal's near-future departure. "That's why he's lived all over the world. He's done a great job helping us out here, but it was always the plan that he'd move on after a couple of months."

Jeremy nodded solemnly.

"I know plenty of great horsemanship instructors," Maya continued, doing her best to add an optimistic inflection to her voice, "and we'll find someone who can work with you and Molly in the spring. How does that sound?"

Lips pressed into a thin line, Jeremy half nodded as he kicked an imaginary stone on the ground.

She turned to her dad, not sure whether to be more upset with him for hiring Cal in the first place, or with herself for allowing him to whittle his way into her and Jeremy's lives. But it was futile to point fingers, she realized. All she could do now was fix the situation before it got worse—and fix it fast.

"Can we talk for a minute?" she asked her dad as she nodded toward the office.

He answered *yes* with his eyes, and together they headed off.

Cal leaned against the back of his truck, wondering what the heck had just happened. Or at least wondered for all of two seconds.

Do you really need to ask?

He closed his eyes, fully realizing that Maya's fears had just unfolded in front of her. Jeremy was looking to him to be someone that he wasn't. A role model. A father figure. His mother's significant other.

But in reality, he was just the "traveling horse vet" who was temporarily filling in until a permanent replacement was found. *Right?*

But if that were true, then why was he feeling so utterly miserable right now? With Maya and her dad holed up in the office, and Jeremy having wandered off to the barn, there was no one around to answer his question.

It's only you, mate.

But wasn't that the story of his life? A story that his actions perpetuated. But recognizing a pattern, and abandoning it for a better alternative, were two different things. *I am who I am.* A defiant declaration that had brought him solace so many times in the past. But not so much right now.

He checked his watch: Two more late-afternoon appointments were about to get underway. He wondered whether to seek out Maya and let her know that he was leaving, but decided to quietly depart. The notion of leaving—regardless of the context—was simply too much of a weighted issue to touch right now.

It was near dusk when he arrived back at the clinic. Spotting Maya's truck in the parking area, he felt the knot in his stomach—first tied when Jeremy had asked about helping with Molly in the spring—flip over itself in a manner that would make a gymnast proud.

Maybe she already forgot about this morning—a thought that he knew should be filed under Wishful Thinking.

"I thought that was you," Maya said as she emerged from the barn, wiping a spot of dirt from her forehead with her sleeve. No confrontation. He was feeling better already. And then, the three most dreaded words known to man.

"Can we talk?"

His smile froze in mid-curve, then slowly deflated. "Sure."

Maya scanned their surroundings, then pointed to a small picnic table to the right of the office.

Cal brushed fallen leaves off the top of the red-stained wooden table as he sat down on the attached bench, more to distract himself from the dread of what was possibly coming than to ensure a clutter-free surface.

Maya sat across from him, her soulful gray eyes looking into his own before casting downward. She took a deep breath and then another, as if gearing up to deliver some news that she knew would not be well received. Finally, she looked back up at him.

"I talked with my dad, and we're going to pay you for the rest of the contract that you signed, but after you finish out this week, we... I mean I...would like you to leave."

She squeezed her eyes shut, as if trying to soften the blow, but whether it was for her sake or his, Cal couldn't tell.

Stunned into silence, he could do little more than stare at Maya in disbelief. He knew she was upset about his exchange with Jeremy earlier that day... but upset enough to show him the door, and with a swift kick in the butt on the way out? *That* he hadn't seen coming.

"Like I said," Maya continued, "you'll be paid in full. My dad and I are both in agreement on this, so no worries there."

"It's not about the money, Maya. I just don't understand—"

"Yes, you do," Maya interjected, eyes determined yet pained at the same time. Her harshness further tightened the knot in his stomach, and added a new obstruction into this throat.

"Jeremy's become attached to you in a way that I hoped wouldn't happen. And I know you're probably thinking you just have a month left on your contract, so why not finish it out. But that would be a month more of him seeing you as someone you're not."

Cal jerked his head back, as though dodging the knife behind her words. But unfortunately, he didn't move fast enough.

"Seeing me as someone I'm not?" Heat rose from his cheeks, searing his brain in the process. Was she implying that he had somehow deceived them as to his true nature? "I've never pretended to be someone other than who I am."

It seemed like such an obvious statement to make. But then again, he knew there were plenty of people in the world who *did* put a false self forward, so perhaps the distinction needed to be made.

"I know, Cal," she conceded, her voice softening. "None of this is anything that you've done wrong. Or deliberately. I want you to know that. But Jeremy sees you as someone in his life—in *our* lives—who's going to continue to be a part of that, and it's just not true. It never was. All I'm doing is trying to lessen the hurt for him." Her eyes, now glossy and vulnerable, met his. "And for me."

"What are you going to do without an extra set of hands?" he asked. It was a filler question as he stalled for time. He needed to process everything, but the gears in his brain were shocked into stupor.

"We've already posted a job ad, this time for a permanent position. That was the plan all along after my dad hired you to fill in temporarily. We just moved up the timetable a bit."

Cal nodded. There were so many questions swirling in his mind, but only one that he gave voice to. "Have you told Jeremy yet?"

"No, but I plan to talk to him tonight. After what happened today, it's not like any of this will be coming out of left field. But I know he's going to have a hard time accepting things."

"I'm so sorry, Maya." She stiffened as his voice

choked up. "It was never my intention to swoop in and turn things upside down for the two of you like this. I care too much to…"

Care too much to what? Maya waited for Cal to say more, but was instead greeted with eyes that were filled with regret. It's not how she wanted his time here to end. *She* cared too much to have him hurt this way.

"It's all going to be okay," she said quietly, gently squeezing his hand as it rested on the table. "Children are more resilient than we sometimes give them credit for. He'll get through this."

"And you?"

Ugh, why did he have to ask this?

From the get-go, Maya's number one concern had been to protect Jeremy. After all, she was an adult who could handle heartbreak, or so she had convinced herself. But clearly she had miscalculated, because right now, her heart was shattered into a million pieces. And she wasn't sure it would ever be whole again.

Her mind raced back to all the opportunities Cal had to say what she so desperately wanted to hear. *I don't want to leave. I want to stay here forever with you. I don't want to run anymore.* But in the end, all he could say was goodbye.

"I'll be okay," she finally said, hoping she only imagined that her voice had just cracked in front of him." And the pained look on Cal's face? Perhaps she was only imagining that, too.

Later that night, Cal felt around on the bed for his phone in the dark, then pressed the side button to illuminate the screen and check the time. It was 2:00 a.m. Three hours of lying awake…and counting.

Jumping from one gig to the next, to one corner of the world and one new set of temporary colleagues and acquaintances…*this* was his jam. And always had been.

But something was different now. It was as if he'd previously sailed through his adult life tossing aside attachments before they even had a chance to form, and now something…or more like *someone*…had stuck. And stuck big.

He stared up the ceiling, fully recognizing that his life was now at a crossroads. He could continue on his usual trajectory, making decisions based solely on his wants and needs. The only problem was… something had shifted inside of him, rendering it impossible to continue thinking of himself as a lone beacon in the night.

It was him, Maya and Jeremy.

But *feeling* something, and living the reality, were two different things. And separating the two? That was one thing known as courage.

CHAPTER FOURTEEN

"I PRINTED OUT some résumés and cover letters that came over," Maria said, handing several sheets of paper to Maya.

Maya grimaced as she leafed through the sparse printouts. "That's it?"

"I know. But we did just post the job. And it's not like there's a ton of available horse vets circulating around."

"Two female candidates and two male." She handed several sheets back to Maria. "No men—I should have mentioned this before we posted the job."

"Maya!" Maria exclaimed incredulously. "You can't do that. It's discrimination."

Maya was just joking…kind of, sort of…but it was worth keeping the ruse going just to see Maria's eye-bulging reaction. "I'm making hiring decisions based on what I know will and won't work. That's not discriminatory."

Maria took off her reading glasses and set them on the desk with an exasperated sigh that was quickly followed with an empathetic smile. "Look, I know what you went through in the aftermath of Max leaving, and your dad filled me in yesterday on your concerns with Cal and Jeremy's attachment to him."

There was something in Maria's kind eyes and tone of voice that told Maya she knew the attachment issue was not Jeremy's alone.

"But you could be missing out on the perfect candidate by outright dismissing all men." She glanced at a sheet of paper, then held it up. "This one, for example, is highly qualified and he's married, so you don't have to worry about him being anything but a professional colleague."

Maya knitted her eyebrows together. "He says that on his résumé?"

"No—in his cover letter. Here, I'll read it to you." Donning her reading glasses once more, she began: "'Dear Sir or Madam…'" She paused to look up at Maya. "I guess you're a madam."

Maya grinned. "I've been called worse."

Maria chuckled, then resumed reading. "'As a board-certified equine veterinarian who has devoted my life to the care and welfare of horses, I read the job posting at Northern Vermont Equine Associates with great interest. Maplewood looks like a wonderful small town for my wife and I to settle down in and raise our family. I believe being a horse vet is more than a career—it's a way of life, and one that my family is fully on board with. I feel confident that I can provide compassionate, expert veterinary care for your equine clients, and I look forward to the chance to share my qualifications with you in person. Sincerely, Jackson Smith.'"

"Hmm."

"Hmm? Does that mean you'll follow up with him?"

Maya knew it was ridiculous to even toy with the idea of automatically disqualifying male vets. After all, what did that say about *her* if she was concerned about becoming romantically involved with another colleague? Did she not have the ability to keep her personal and professional lives separate?

Of course I can do that, she silently acknowledged. The problem was, she hadn't. But that was on her...and there was no reason why she couldn't learn from her mistakes. She thought she had after the Max fiasco, but then Cal came into her life and snuck into her heart...

Maya squeezed her eyes shut, as if doing so could catapult Cal from her thoughts and feelings. But he was still too much a part of both.

As if she needed a reminder of this—which she didn't—the office door opened and Cal stepped inside. He did a double take upon seeing Maya, which she returned in full.

"I need to check on some supplies for reorder," Maria said unconvincingly as she rose from her desk. "I'll be back in a few." She smiled a little too knowingly in both their directions before heading out of the office.

Cal waited for the door to close behind her, then

turned to Maya. "I just came by to sign an amended contract." He glanced at the résumés in her hand, then looked back up at her, his expressionless face giving away little. "How's the job search going?"

Maya wished it wasn't so easy for him to ask about his replacement, as though his leaving was simply business as usual. But wasn't that his MO to begin with?

"Only four candidates so far, but it's still early," Maya replied, doing her best not to look too deeply into his eyes. A good thing to practice, given that soon Cal—and his dreamy eyes—would be firmly planted on another continent.

"Anyone good?"

She debated whether to give him the full rundown. Two candidates just out of veterinary college, but both referring to the position in their cover letters as a "first step" in their careers, which hardly boded well for longevity. Still, that didn't entirely rule them out. And two more established candidates, one who felt the need to disclose his marital status in his cover letter—perhaps to paint himself as family friendly and with small-town values—and the other who was "looking for a change after being micromanaged for too many years." *Oomph.*

She opted for a quick and truthful summary. "There are a couple of promising prospects."

Cal's smile was tight, his voice pleasant enough yet more terse than usual. "Glad to hear it."

"What about you? Are things moving ahead with the job in England?"

He nodded. "I've had a couple of Zoom calls, and the next step is an in-person interview."

An in-person interview. In England...three thousand miles away...an insurmountable ocean and unnavigable circumstances between them.

The energy required for Maya to maintain a smile through these thoughts was enough to propel her through a twenty-mile marathon. *And I'm not even a runner.* Still, she did her best to appear happy for him. "That's great. Well, good luck with that."

"Maya…"

She waited for him to say more. When he didn't, she realized that maybe it was just as well. After all, what could he possibly say at this point? *Sorry that I broke your heart. Take care and have a nice life!*

"I said goodbye to Jeremy earlier," Cal finally said after a prolonged silence.

Maya gave the slightest nod. "He told me." She wouldn't share the part about Jeremy crying to her as he did. "Well, good luck with everything," she said, her voice cracking slightly before she could finish the forced sentiment. She looked at the office door, hoping he'd take the hint. He did.

And so, moments later, he silently walked out of the door—and her life—for good.

CHAPTER FIFTEEN

MAYA STOOD OUTSIDE the clinic office and cupped her hands over her eyes to shield them from the midday sun. In the distance, she could see the tiny white speck of a passenger jet as it made its way across the sky.

Was Cal possibly on board, heading to his next adventure? It was Wednesday—five days since his official last day at the practice. They hadn't spoken since their awkward parting of ways in Maria's office, so she could only assume he was en route to England—or already there.

Inside the office once again, she sat in Maria's chair behind the desk, nervously tapping the butt of a pen on a desk pad. She didn't have much experience interviewing job candidates, but that wasn't the only reason she was struggling to focus. Images of Cal incessantly flooded her mind. Would she ever get over him? It simply didn't seem possible.

A knock on the slightly ajar door pulled her from her thoughts. "Come on in," she said in as friendly a voice as she could muster up.

The candidate did as instructed, entering the room and taking a seat across from Maya.

Ping!

The pen dropped out of her hand and bounced off her open laptop. "Cal! What are you doing here?"

A grin slowly spread across his face. "Nice to see you, too."

She had so many questions that it was impossible to get even one off the ground. "I'm about to interview someone for the vet position any second now."

"I know."

"How do you…?" Her question was cut short, in part because her gaping mouth refused to cooperate. *No…it can't be*.

Cal leaned forward and extended his hand. "Jackson Smith. Nice to meet you."

"Hold on a minute." She leaned forward and held her head in her hands, as if worried that it might topple off due to shock. Then she picked up the résumé and cover letter, flapping it in the air. "Are you saying this has been *you* all along?"

Cal's already expansive grin further widened to the point that Maya wondered if the corner of his lips would soon meet at the back of his head. "Yup."

She glanced at the cover letter, her hands trembling. "So all of this is one big lie?"

Cal teetered his head from side to side. "Ehhh… not exactly."

"Well, your name isn't Jackson Smith—let's start with that."

"Jackson's my middle name."

"And Smith?"

"Okay, that one's a fib. But it's generic enough

that I figured I probably have an ancestor or two by that name, if you go back far enough."

Maya's heart was now racing so hard that she was convinced her chest must be visibly pulsating. "And you're married and want to raise a family in Maplewood." *Let's see how he talks his way out of this concoction*, she thought pointedly.

Cal stared at her. And stared some more. "Not a lie." He paused, "At least I hope not."

If Maya's head could swivel 360 degrees, it'd be twirling like a top. But since it had to conform to the laws of physics, she continued to look straight at him, her eyes deeply perplexed. "Cal… I am so confused right now. Can you please tell me what the heck is going on?"

"Maya, I wrote that cover letter imagining what I hope I can say about myself…about *us*…in the very near future."

Maya wanted to say, *Of course, now I understand!* Except that she didn't. Because it *almost* sounded like he was implying that she was the wife, and together with Jeremy, the three of them were the family. But that couldn't be what he meant… *could it*?

"I've been doing a lot of thinking this past week. *A lot*. And I've come to realize that in so many ways, my life has been a cliché."

Between her widened eyes and über-raised eyebrows, Maya looked like she'd been zapped by a cattle prod. "A cliché?" she repeated tepidly.

"The young boy tossed around from one foster home to another, never feeling like he was truly loved. So he spends his adult life reenacting that very same pattern, never sticking around one place too long to form real relationships. That is, until he meets an amazing woman who makes him see everything in a whole new light."

It took several moments for a slightly stunned Maya to form a reply. "Have you been binge-watching *Dr. Phil* or something?"

Cal chuckled. "I know—I kind of scared myself with the way I've been self-analyzing things. But that's what love will make you do."

Oh boy...

Maya felt like she could melt into the chair, but that wasn't going to happen. Not when Cal had already walked around the desk and pulled her up into his arms. "I love you, Maya Evans. And I want to spend my life with you and Jeremy."

"I love you, too," Maya said, her voice as stunned as the rest of her. Could this actually be happening? It seemed too good...too unbelievable...to be true, but reality came crashing back in the best way possible as Cal pulled her into a passionate kiss.

"I do have a question," she said once they finally came up for air. "Why didn't you just say from the get-go that you wanted to stay, rather than send a résumé pretending to be someone else?"

"I could have," he conceded. "But wasn't this surprise more fun?" As Maya laughed, he added, "Plus,

I was working on a few things behind the scenes, and I wanted to make sure everything was in place before the big reveal."

Maya's stomach butterflies began to dance again. "What big reveal?"

Cal's grin returned full force. "Let's take a drive to your place."

Fifteen minutes later, Cal pulled his truck into Maya's driveway.

"Who are all these people at my place?" she asked, eyes scanning a small crowd spread out in front of the porch.

"Friends who are here to help."

Maya's confusion was growing exponentially. "I don't think I have this many friends," she said frankly. Truth was, she had never been a social butterfly, flitting from one superficial friendship to the next, but more like a reserved caterpillar who clung tightly to several long-held, cherished friendships. And yet, she estimated the group mingling just in front of the open porch to be at least fifteen individuals.

"Cal, *what* is going on?"

"Come on," he said with a grin as he nodded toward the group. "Let's go find out."

As they walked hand in hand, familiar faces began to come into view. Some were clients, others were their spouses whom she'd met on occasion during vet calls.

Cal gestured to the group. "Maya, I'd like you to

meet the *new* Happy Hooves Horse Rescue operations team."

"I'm not sure I understand what's going on here."

"Well—and don't get upset with Maria for this—but I talked her into sharing the Equine Associates mailing list with me. Last week, I sent out an email asking for volunteers to help get the barn and fencing in working order. Everyone's here to help make your dream…" He reached over and squeezed her hand, then called to Jeremy, who'd been standing in front of a smiling Gus, his hands clasping both of his grandson's shoulders. Jeremy quickly trotted over, his cheeks nearly bursting with an outsize smile. "To make *our* dream, as a family, for a horse sanctuary come true."

"I don't believe this," Maya murmured in sheer awe. "Is this really happening?"

Clapping and cheers ensued as Cal leaned over and kissed her on the cheek. "It most definitely is." He leaned in further to whisper in her ear: "I'm keeping it G-rated for the all-ages audience, but get those soft, beautiful lips ready for when we're alone later."

I've now officially died and gone to heaven. Though Cal's strong arm around her side, propping her happy-shaky body upward, confirmed that she was still very much amongst the living.

Cal pointed to a burly man with a thick beard, who stood across the way. "We have an electrician…"

"Hi, I'm Rick."

"He's with me," Georgette, a longtime client who raised miniature horses, said with a laugh.

"And a roofer," Cal continued.

"I'm Mike, Janice's son. And I brought along a couple of my roofing buddies. This is Craig and Dave."

Maya hoped everyone could see the immense gratitude in her eyes as she nodded in their direction with an unbridled smile, because at the moment, words escaped her.

"We also have a special guest of honor today," Cal said as he pointed to Cathy. Standing next to her sister, she waved to Maya. "Once I kick the crap out of this cancer, I'll be back here to visit everyone. And I can't wait."

That's it. I can't hold it together anymore. As Maya began to cry, Cal pulled her in even closer. She looked up at him, only to find that his own glossy eyes were just barely holding back tears. "It takes a village," he said quietly.

"True," she said softly. "But there wouldn't be this village if it weren't for one incredibly special man who made it happen. I love you."

He smiled. "I love you, too." Defying his G-rated promise, he kissed her on the lips, a long, lingering smooch that prompted another wave of applause from the crowd.

"Come on," he said to Jeremy as he tousled his hair. "Let's go pick out the perfect stall for Molly."

Holding onto Jeremy's hand, he reached out and grasped Maya's hand as well.

And with that, the trio headed to the barn. Together...like the family they were always meant to be.

* * * * *

*If you enjoyed this story,
check out this other great read from
Tessa Scott*
Healing the Baby Surgeon's Heart
Available now!

Get up to 4 Free Books!

We'll send you 2 free books from each series you try PLUS a free Mystery Gift.

Both the **Harlequin Presents** and **Harlequin Medical Romance** series feature exciting stories of passion and drama.

YES! Please send me 2 FREE novels from Harlequin Presents or Harlequin Medical Romance and my FREE gift (gift is worth about $10 retail). After receiving them, if I don't wish to receive any more books, I can return the shipping statement marked "cancel." If I don't cancel, I will receive 6 brand-new larger-print novels every month and be billed just $7.19 each in the U.S., or $7.99 each in Canada, or 4 brand-new Harlequin Medical Romance Larger-Print books every month and be billed just $7.19 each in the U.S. or $7.99 each in Canada, a savings of 20% off the cover price. It's quite a bargain! Shipping and handling is just 50¢ per book in the U.S. and $1.25 per book in Canada.* I understand that accepting the 2 free books and gift places me under no obligation to buy anything. I can always return a shipment and cancel at any time. The free books and gift are mine to keep no matter what I decide.

Choose one:
- ☐ **Harlequin Presents Larger-Print** (176/376 BPA G36Y)
- ☐ **Harlequin Medical Romance** (171/371 BPA G36Y)
- ☐ **Or Try Both!** (176/376 & 171/371 BPA G36Z)

Name (please print)

Address   Apt. #

City   State/Province   Zip/Postal Code

Email: Please check this box ☐ if you would like to receive newsletters and promotional emails from Harlequin Enterprises ULC and its affiliates. You can unsubscribe anytime.

Mail to the Harlequin Reader Service:
IN U.S.A.: P.O. Box 1341, Buffalo, NY 14240-8531
IN CANADA: P.O. Box 603, Fort Erie, Ontario L2A 5X3

Want to explore our other series or interested in ebooks? Visit www.ReaderService.com or call 1-800-873-8635.

---

*Terms and prices subject to change without notice. Prices do not include sales taxes, which will be charged (if applicable) based on your state or country of residence. Canadian residents will be charged applicable taxes. Offer not valid in Quebec. This offer is limited to one order per household. Books received may not be as shown. Not valid for current subscribers to the Harlequin Presents or Harlequin Medical Romance series. All orders subject to approval. Credit or debit balances in a customer's account(s) may be offset by any other outstanding balance owed by or to the customer. Please allow 4 to 6 weeks for delivery. Offer available while quantities last.

Your Privacy—Your information is being collected by Harlequin Enterprises ULC, operating as Harlequin Reader Service. For a complete summary of the information we collect, how we use this information and to whom it is disclosed, please visit our privacy notice located at https://corporate.harlequin.com/privacy-notice. Notice to California Residents – Under California law, you have specific rights to control and access your data. For more information on these rights and how to exercise them, visit https://corporate.harlequin.com/california-privacy. For additional information for residents of other U.S. states that provide their residents with certain rights with respect to personal data, visit https://corporate.harlequin.com/other-state-residents-privacy-rights/.

HPHM25